Model Child Care Health Policies

5th Edition

Susan S. Aronson, MD, FAAP
Editor

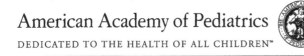

American Academy of Pediatrics
DEDICATED TO THE HEALTH OF ALL CHILDREN™

Pennsylvania Chapter

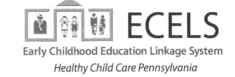

ECELS
Early Childhood Education Linkage System
Healthy Child Care Pennsylvania

American Academy of Pediatrics Department of Marketing and Publications

Maureen DeRosa, MPA, Director, Department of Marketing and Publications

Mark Grimes, Director, Division of Product Development

Eileen Glasstetter, MS, Manager, Product Development

Carrie Peters, Editorial Assistant

Sandi King, MS, Director, Division of Publishing and Production Services

Shannan Martin, Publishing and Production Services Specialist

Jason Crase, Manager, Editorial Services

Linda Diamond, Manager, Art Direction and Production

Julia Lee, Director, Division of Marketing and Sales

Linda Smessaert, MSIMC, Brand Manager, Clinical and Professional Publications

Suggested Citation: Pennsylvania Chapter of the American Academy of Pediatrics. *Model Child Care Health Policies.* Aronson SS, ed. 5th ed. Elk Grove Village, IL: American Academy of Pediatrics; 2014. www.ecels-healthychildcarepa.org

Library of Congress Control Number: 2013939547
ISBN: 978-1-58110-826-2
eISBN: 978-1-58110-830-9
MA0689

The recommendations in this publication do not indicate an exclusive course of treatment or serve as a standard of medical care. Variations, taking into account individual circumstances, may be appropriate.

Products are mentioned for informational purposes only. Inclusion in this publication does not imply endorsement by the American Academy of Pediatrics. The American Academy of Pediatrics is not responsible for the content of the resources mentioned in this publication. Web site addresses are as current as possible but may change at any time.

The publishers have made every effort to trace the copyright holders for borrowed material. If they have inadvertently overlooked any, they will be pleased to make the necessary arrangements at first opportunity.

Printed in the United States of America.

9-342/rep0818

4 5 6 7 8 9 10

Reviewers/Contributors

Abbey Alkon, RN, PNP, PhD
Professor
Department of Family Health Care Nursing
University of California, San Francisco,
    School of Nursing
Director
California Childcare Health Program
San Francisco, CA

Nancy Alleman, RN, BSN, CRNP, CSN
Lead Training/Technical Assistance Coordinator
Early Childhood Education Linkage System
Pennsylvania Chapter, American Academy of Pediatrics
Media, PA

Beth Baker, MS (Counseling and Human Relations)
Family Services Director
Children's Village
Philadelphia, PA

Sandra Cianciolo, MPH, RN
National Training Institute for Child Care Health
    Consultants
Department of Maternal and Child Health
Gillings School of Global Public Health
University of North Carolina at Chapel Hill
Chapel Hill, NC

Jean M. Cimino, MPH
Content Comanager, *Caring for Our Children,*
    3rd Edition
National Resource Center for Health and Safety
    in Child Care and Early Education
University of Colorado College of Nursing
Aurora, CO

Patricia S. Cole, MPH
Senior Director
Indiana Accreditation Project
Indiana Association for the Education
    of Young Children
Indianapolis, IN

Judy L. Collins, MS
Licensing Consultant
Norman, OK

Angela A. Crowley, PhD, APRN, PNP-BC, FAAN
Associate Professor
Yale University School of Nursing
New Haven, CT

Beth A. DelConte, MD, FAAP
Pediatric Advisor
Early Childhood Education Linkage System
Pennsylvania Chapter, American Academy of Pediatrics
Media, PA

Steven B. Eng, MPH, CIPHI(C)
Manager, Strategic and Operations Support
Health Protection
Fraser Health
Port Moody, BC
Canada

Kathleen M. Ford, RN, BC
Child Care Health Consultation Systems Coordinator
Nurse Manager Child Care Nurse Consultation
Pima County Public Health Nursing
Pima County Health Department
Tucson, AZ

Danette S. Glassy, MD, FAAP
Cochair of the Steering Committee for
    Caring for Our Children, 3rd Edition
Chairperson, American Academy of Pediatrics
    Section on Early Education and Child Care
Pediatrician, Mercer Island Pediatrics
Mercer Island, WA

Barbara U. Hamilton, MA
Early Care and Education Specialist
Division of Home Visiting and Early Childhood Systems
Maternal and Child Health Bureau
Rockville, MD

Rosemary Johnston, RN, BSN, MSN
Training and Technical Assistance Coordinator
Early Childhood Education Linkage System
Pennsylvania Chapter, American Academy of Pediatrics
Media, PA

Marilyn J. Krajicek, EdD, RN, FAAN
University of Colorado College of Nursing
Director, National Resource Center for Health and
   Safety in Child Care and Early Education
Aurora, CO

Nikki Lee, RN, BSN, MS, IBCLC, CCE, CIMI, ANLC, CKC
Elkins Park, PA

Patti Lucarelli, MSN, RN-BC, CPNP, APN
Pediatric Nurse Practitioner
Jersey Shore University Medical Center
Jane H. Booker Family Health Center
Neptune, NJ

Janice C. Maker, BSN, MS, CRNP
Child Care Health Consultant
McMurray, PA

**Aleksandra (Sandy) McDonnell, MSN, RN, CRNP,
   PNP-BC**
Child Care Health Consultant
Program Director, EPIC: Pediatric Obesity Evaluation,
   Treatment and Prevention in Community Settings
Pennsylvania Chapter, American Academy of Pediatrics
Media, PA

Sarah Myers, RN
Child Care Health Consultant
National Training Institute for Child Care Health
   Consultants (graduate and child care health
   consultant trainer)
North Dakota Child Care Resource & Referral
Fargo, ND

Elizabeth (Betsy) L. M. Miller, BSN, RN, BC
Child Care Health & Safety, LLC
Newtown Square, PA

Mary Anne Miller, RN, MPH, CHES
Child Care Health Consultant
Adjunct Professor Health Care Administration
Stonehill College
Easton, MA

Stephanie Olmore, MA
Director, Quality Enhancements Initiative
National Association for the Education
   of Young Children
Washington, DC

Robert P. Olympia, MD, FAAP
Associate Professor, Emergency Medicine and Pediatrics
Penn State College of Medicine
Attending Physician, Department of Emergency
   Medicine
Penn State Milton S. Hershey Medical Center
Penn State Children's Hospital
Hershey, PA

Amy Requa, MSN, CRNP
Health Consultant
State Oral Health Coordinator
Pennsylvania Head Start Association
Harrisburg, PA

Judith Rex, RN, BC, MSN
Director, Healthcare Education
Northampton Community College
Bethlehem, PA

Bobbie Rose, RN, PHN
Child Care Health Consultant
University of California, San Francisco
California Childcare Health Program
San Francisco, CA

Linda Satkowiak, ND, RN, CNS, NCSN
Content Comanager, *Caring for Our Children,*
   3rd Edition
National Resource Center for Health and Safety
   in Child Care and Early Education
University of Colorado College of Nursing
Aurora, CO

Jeanne M. VanOrsdal, MEd
Manager, Early Education and Child Care Initiatives
American Academy of Pediatrics
Elk Grove Village, IL

Additional Assistance
The staff members of the PA AAP program, the Early
Childhood Education Linkage System–Healthy Child
Care Pennsylvania, have contributed their experience in
the field to make this and all previous editions as useful
as possible.

Table of Contents

Section 3 13
Planned Program, Teaching, and Guidance

Section 4 19
Nutrition, Food Handling, and Feeding

Section 8 51
Environmental Health

Appendixes

Introduction

Sources for This Edition

The fifth edition of *Model Child Care Health Policies* (MCCHP) is a tool to foster adoption and implementation of best practices for health and safety in group care settings for young children. These settings include early care and education as well as before- and after-school child care programs. It is the product of broad and ongoing input from key leaders representing multiple organizations and agencies over many years. In 1991, the Pennsylvania Chapter of the American Academy of Pediatrics (PA AAP) reviewed policies submitted by more than 100 child care programs (centers and family child care homes) as part of a study conducted by the Early Childhood Education Linkage System (ECELS), a program of the PA AAP. From these, ECELS selected the best practice policies for specific topics and edited, merged, and published these as the first edition of MCCHP. In 1992, ECELS reviewed and contributed to recommendations for written health policies in the first edition of the widely used reference *Caring for Our Children: National Health and Safety Performance Standards: Guidelines for Out-of-Home Child Care Programs*. This national reference was authored by the American Public Health Association and American Academy of Pediatrics and funded by a grant from the Maternal and Child Health Bureau of the Health Resources and Services Administration, US Department of Health and Human Services.

The Early Childhood Education Linkage System prepared subsequent editions, including this fifth edition, of MCCHP by drawing on comments and suggestions from users as well as standards in the then-current editions of *Caring for Our Children*. The third edition of *Caring for Our Children*, retitled *Caring for Our Children: National Health and Safety Performance Standards: Guidelines for Early Care and Education Programs*, was published in 2011 and served as the source for standards in the preparation of this edition of MCCHP.[1] In the rest of this text, the third edition of *Caring for Our Children* is referred to as *CFOC3*.

Reviews and adaptations prepared by technical experts, child care health consultants (CCHCs), early education and child care directors, and other users have been particularly helpful in the revision process. While the fifth edition of MCCHP draws on the foundation of the fourth edition, most of the text has been rewritten. Attributing individual concepts, items, and phrases within the text would reduce the readability of this edition. Instead, this update of MCCHP acknowledges the following contributions made by some reviewers of their model policies:

- Arizona (2006; sent by Kathleen M. Ford, RN, BC, child care health consultation systems coordinator, Nurse Manager Child Care Nurse Consultation, Pima County Public Health Nursing, Pima County Health Department, Tucson, AZ; www.pimahealth.org/pubhealthnursing/documents/CCHCmanual_WEBFULL.pdf).
- California (2005 and ongoing updates by Abbey Alkon, RN, PNP, PhD, professor, University of California, San Francisco School of Nursing; director, California Childcare Health Program, and Bobbie Rose, RN, PHN, San Francisco, CA; www.ucsfchildcarehealth.org).
- Indiana (2006; sent by Patricia S. Cole, MPH, past program coordinator, Indiana Child Care Health Consultant Program; www.in.gov/fssa/carefinder/2750.htm; currently senior director, Indiana Accreditation Project, Indiana Association for the Education of Young Children, Inc, Indianapolis).
- The National Training Institute for Child Care Health Consultants at the University of North Carolina, Chapel Hill (2013; materials on policy development and individual topics accessed in password-protected CCHC trainer tool kits; http://nti.unc.edu).
- Seattle-King County, Washington (2006–2009; recommended by Danette S. Glassy, MD, FAAP, cochair of the Steering Committee for *CFOC3*; www.kingcounty.gov/healthservices/health/child/childcare/modelhealth.aspx).
- Significant individual contributions to this edition were made by the reviewers listed in the front matter of MCCHP.

Many of the policies in this fifth edition of MCCHP paraphrase the wording in one or more *CFOC3* standards; this is indicated by a superscript reference to the standard, eg, *CFOC3* Std. 2.1.1.7. In a few places, the standard is directly quoted;

this is indicated by quotation marks around *CFOC3* text. Users will find it helpful to review these referenced standards. Each of the standards in *CFOC3* includes the standard itself, the rationale for the standard, comments about implementation of the standard, and references to the evidence in the scientific literature that justifies the standard.

What Is a Child Care Health Policy?

A *child care health policy* is a statement of what the program intends to do about any aspect of the program that affects the health (well-being) of children and adults who are involved with it. Minimally, it should address program compliance with applicable regulations. Better, it should describe the commitment of the program to best practice, as indicated in *CFOC3*. Optimally, it should describe performance that the program achieves. A policy might specify intended compliance with accreditation standards, such as those of the National Association for the Education of Young Children (NAEYC) (www.naeyc.org) for center-based care or the National Association for Family Child Care (www.nafcc.org) for non-parental care of up to 12 children in the home of teacher(s)/caregiver(s). Policies should be explicit and measurable. They are not goals; they define expected performance.

Use of *Model Child Care Health Policies*

Since the fourth edition of MCCHP was published in 2002, more than 20,000 copies have been distributed by NAEYC. Users include health professionals who provide technical assistance, professional development (training) and consultation, agency staff who ensure compliance and promote quality, and providers of group care programs for children. Child care programs of any type can use MCCHP by selecting relevant issues for their operation and modifying the wording to make the selected policies appropriate to the specific setting. These settings include early education and child care centers, small and large family child care homes, part-day programs, child care programs for children who are ill, facilities that serve children with special needs, school-age child care facilities, and drop-in facilities. The model policies in this booklet can be adapted for public, private, Head Start, and tuition-funded facilities.

Each type of program has certain requirements that apply to that specific program that may differ from those another program must meet. For example, Head Start must comply with the published Head Start Performance Standards such as the specifications found in 45 CFR 1304 (Child Health and Development), 45 CFR 1308 (Disabilities) and 45 CFR 1310 (Transportation). The health and safety topics in these Head Start Performance Standards are addressed in this edition of MCCHP. Many facilities are regulated by state, county, or municipal agencies. Government regulations are the legal floor below which a program is not allowed to operate. The specific regulatory requirements vary from one state, county, or municipality to another. The National Association of Child Care Resource & Referral Agencies/Child Care Aware of America (NACCRRA) reports that all states include health and safety in their licensing and compliance regulations.[2,3]

All of the most commonly covered health and safety topics NACCRRA found in state regulations are included in MCCHP. Be sure to check the wording of local or state regulations for each policy topic and include compliance with the intent of the legal requirement in your site-specific policies.

Centers and family child care homes can have policies and practices that go beyond regulations—and do so often. Standards describe expected performance, usually intended to be used to measure whether operations meet a defined threshold of quality. Recommendations and guidance are usually based on expert advice about how to perform. Measurability is a key test for standards, recommendations, guidance or regulatory requirements, and site-specific policies. The most implementable statements are those that are clear and measurable. Users must know when they have met or are not meeting expected performance.

Policies should be living documents. Problems that occur in the operation of a program identify a need for new policies or revision of old policies. Site-specific adaptation of these model policies should reflect the solution the program chooses to use. Policies are tools to communicate expectations of the program to new and existing staff members, consultants, visitors, and families who have enrolled or are considering enrolling their children.

Developing Site-Specific Health and Safety Policies

These model policies are intended to ease the burden of writing site-specific health and safety policies from scratch. They cover a wide range of aspects of operation of early education and child care programs. Users are expected to select, adapt, or adopt portions that they think are helpful in their programs. Professionals who provide technical assistance and professional development for child care programs can help directors and other staff members choose which model policies to work on and how to adjust them to fit their site-specific requirements. Many of the model policies provide blanks to fill in site-specific information with cue words about what to insert in the blank.

When a new policy is being drafted or when a change in policy is contemplated, be sure to invite input from those who will be affected by the policy, those who have expertise to bear on the policy, and those who have the authority and responsibility for making sure the policy is followed. Then, after considering the input, be sure to inform everyone involved about what change was made and the rationale for adopting or rejecting any input. One of the experts to involve in the process should be a licensed health professional who serves in an ongoing relationship with the program staff as the facility's CCHC. Current evidence shows that multiple CCHC site visits over the course of a year coupled with ongoing accessibility of the CCHC is associated with quality improvement of the program and desired child outcomes.[4-6] Programs that serve children younger than 3 years should have at least monthly CCHC visits. The CCHC should be a health professional with general knowledge of health and safety in child care facilities. Programs that serve children who are between 3 and 5 years of age should have at least quarterly health consultant visits. Programs that serve school-aged children should have at least 2 visits a year. Family child care home networks and individual family child care homes should strive for the same frequency of visits related to the age group served. The frequency of visits should meet the needs of the children who are enrolled and of the program staff for professional development and support. During these visits, the health consultant's observations and collaborative planning for improvement should include measures to prevent infectious diseases and injury, safe sleep practices, nutrition, oral health, physical activity, emergency preparedness, medication administration, and the care of children with special needs. Documentation of the dates and content of these visits should be kept in the facility's files.[CFOC3 Std. 1.6.0.2] Arrange for the CCHC to review the policies when they are being created, when an incident or injury occurs, and at least annually. Each policy should include the date of the most recent review. Be sure they are updated or reaffirmed at least annually.[CFOC3 Std. 9.2.3.17] Have an attorney review the policies when they are new or revised. These professionals have the expertise to advise the program about adopting current best practice and legal implications of a proposed policy.

A CCHC with overall understanding of health and safety issues is likely to be a pediatric nurse, nurse practitioner, or pediatrician. For some topics such as emergency preparedness, food preparation, or environmental health, health and safety professionals with specialized expertise in those topics may be better suited to do that part of the review. The general CCHC should be a licensed health professional with the necessary knowledge and skills in pediatrics, community health, and care of children in group settings. Some may have prior education or experience in the CCHC role.[CFOC3 Stds. 1.6.0.1, 1.6.0.2] For some matters, the consultant should be an early childhood mental health consultant[CFOC3 Std. 1.6.0.3] or an early childhood education consultant.[CFOC3 Std. 1.6.0.4] Federal support for states to develop systems to educate and deploy CCHCs has been helpful. To locate needed consultants, early education and child care programs can contact public health departments, resource and referral agencies, state child care quality improvement systems, individual health care professionals, or institutions such as children's hospitals, health professional organizations, and universities. For more details about working with a CCHC, see www.healthychildcare.org/WorkWithHP.html.

Consider any costs, barriers, or burdens that might be involved in implementing each policy. For policies to be implemented, they must be reviewed, understood, and thought feasible to those expected to follow them. Staff members and families should be aware of the rationale for policies that apply to them. To support accountability when policies are not followed, everyone expected to follow certain policies needs to have an opportunity to go over them with someone who can review the expectation and reason for each relevant policy. It is easier to deal with noncompliance if everyone has signed a document that indicates they agree to abide by the named list of policies that are relevant to their role in the program.

Once adopted, policies should be available where it is easy for everyone who is expected to comply to access them. Give the list and location of relevant current policies to each family at the time of enrollment and to prospective staff members before hiring them. Invite them to ask questions about any policy that is unclear or causes them concern. If anyone has difficulty reading the written policies or is not fluent in the language in which the policies are written, arrange to go over each relevant policy verbally in a language that is understood.

Format and Vocabulary for Model Policies

For convenience, model policies often use the term *families* to identify parents, legal guardians, and other responsible relatives who care for children. In some situations in which consent is required, the term *parent or legal guardian* indicates the narrower legal focus. This text uses people-first wording when describing specific roles, special needs, or conditions. For example, a policy may be said to apply to a "child with a chronic illness" rather than to a "chronically ill child." The term *teacher/caregiver* includes all adults directly involved in the education and care of children, whether paid or volunteer, or part-time or full-time. The term *staff member* includes all adults who work in any capacity in the facility under the supervision of the person responsible for the operation of the program.

Each model policy has the following components that should be retained in the site-specific policy adapted from it:

- **Title/subject** of the policy
- **Rationale** (ie, why the policy is necessary; related national health and safety standards in *CFOC3* that inform the policy and provide rationale and references as evidence for it)
- **Required action/who is responsible/how communicated** (ie, what, who, where, how, when, including how those affected by the policy will be informed of it)

Help to Improve and Update *Model Child Care Health Policies*

Please send ECELS your suggestions about how the next edition of MCCHP could be made more useful. Let us know how you are using these policies. We look forward to hearing from you and wish you well in your efforts to improve the quality of child care. We will post updates on the ECELS Web site, www.ecels-healthychildcarepa.org, and announce each posting of an update in an e-mail alert from ECELS. To receive e-mail alerts from ECELS, sign up on the home page of the ECELS Web site at www.ecels-healthychildcarepa.org.

Susan S. Aronson, MD, FAAP
Pennsylvania Chapter, American Academy of Pediatrics
Author/Editor, *Model Child Care Health Policies,* 5th Edition
ECELS-Healthy Child Care PA
1400 N Providence Road
Rose Tree Media Corporate Center II, Suite 3007
Media, PA 19063-2043
800/24-ECELS (in PA only)
484/446-3003
E-mail: ecels@paaap.org
Web site: www.ecels-healthychildcarepa.org

References

1. American Academy of Pediatrics, American Public Health Association, National Resource Center for Health and Safety in Child Care and Early Education. *Caring for Our Children: National Health and Safety Performance Standards: Guidelines for Early Care and Education Programs.* 3rd ed. Elk Grove Village, IL: American Academy of Pediatrics; 2011

2. Child Care Aware of America. Child care in America: 2012 state fact sheets. http://www.naccrra.org/sites/default/files/default_site_pages/2012/2012nationalsummaryfactsheets.pdf. Accessed August 28, 2013

3. National Association of Child Care Resource & Referral Agencies. *Leaving Children to Chance: NACCRRA's Ranking of State Standards and Oversight for Small Family Child Care Homes: 2012 Update.* Arlington, VA: National Association of Child Care Resource & Referral Agencies; 2012. http://www.naccrra.org/sites/default/files/default_site_pages/2012/lcc_report_full_april2012.pdf. Accessed August 28, 2013

4. Alkon A, Bernzweig J, To K, Wolff M, Mackie JF. Child care health consultation improves health and safety policies and practices. *Acad Pediatr.* 2009;9(5):366–370

5. Snohomish Health District Child Care Health Program. Child care health consultation: evidence based effectiveness. http://www.napnap.org/docs/CCS_SIG_Evidence_%20Based_%20CCHP.pdf. Accessed August 28, 2013

6. Heath JM. *Creating a Statewide System of Multi-Disciplinary Consultation for Early Care and Education in Connecticut: April 2005.* Farmington, CT: Child Health and Development Institute of Connecticut, Inc; 2005. http://www.chdi.org/admin/uploads/532072684a0c62636a110.pdf. Accessed August 28, 2013

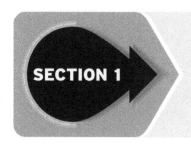

Admission/Enrollment/Attendance

Rationale

- Families and child care staff members must mutually understand and commit to working as partners in the child's care. All those involved in the child's care should be as well-informed as possible before the decision is made to share care of the child with the staff of the child care program and with whoever else will be in the facility when the child is there.

- The program staff members, family, and child will fare best in their ongoing relationship if everyone is prepared for a smooth transfer of responsibility for the child's care. The program should have written documentation of current information about the child and family pertinent to the child's care.

- To provide continuity of care for the child between the program and home and to be sure that each child is accounted for at all times, families and staff members must communicate every day about who is present or unexpectedly absent and about events and changes in routine for the child, the child's family, and the program on a need-to-know basis.

Required Action/Who Is Responsible/How Communicated

A. Admission (Information Gathering by Family and Program to Plan for Child's Care)

1. **Diversity:**

_____
NAME AND ADDRESS OF FACILITY

admits children from the ages of _____ to _____ without regard to race, culture, ethnicity,
AGE   AGE

sex, religion, national origin, ancestry, special health needs, developmental or behavioral concerns, or disabilities. The curriculum reflects respect for different cultures, without stereotyping of any culture.[CFOC3 Std. 2.1.1.8] Program staff members try to communicate in the language best understood by the family. If that language is not spoken English or the family does not understand written English, the program will find a trusted adult who uses the family's language to translate for the family. In addition, the program will suggest ways for family members to communicate with program staff when the program does not have a translator available. For example, the program may help the family to identify a bilingual person in the family's community who can write out the family's communication in English and translate notes that the program writes in English for the family. Staff members will provide opportunities for the child to learn English.[CFOC3 Std. 2.1.1.7]

2. **Review and Signing of Program Policies:** The child's parent/legal guardian and

---

ROLE OF THE STAFF MEMBER WHO IS RESPONSIBLE FOR ADMISSIONS

will review and discuss program policies applicable to the family. Then the parent/legal guardian and

---

TITLE/NAME OF STAFF MEMBER

will sign a document that indicates the review was completed and the content was accepted.

a. **Special Needs:** When the parent or legal guardian of a child identifies that a child has special needs,

---

NAME OF PROGRAM DIRECTOR

and the parent or legal guardian will meet to review the child's requirements for care. The program accepts children for whom the facility is equipped or can be equipped to provide care[CFOC3 Std. 5.1.1.4] and staff members can provide a safe, supportive environment.[CFOC3 Stds. 1.3.2.2, 1.4, 1.6.0.1, 2.1.1, 2.3.3.2, 3.5, 8.2, 8.7, 9.2, 9.4, 10.3.4.5, 10.3.4.6] Program decisions about accepting children with special needs are consistent with the requirements of the Americans with Disabilities Act.[CFOC3 Stds. 8.2.0.1, 8.2.0.2]

NAME OF PROGRAM DIRECTOR

will work with the parent/legal guardian to find a suitable environment for the child if the program is unable to accommodate the child's needs because the needs pose an undue burden as defined by federal law. The child's needs will be specified in a care plan completed by the child's health care professional(s) or in the Individual Family Service Plan/Individual Education Plan.

3. **Admission Agreement:**

a. **Individual Agreement for Each Child:**

TITLE/NAME OF STAFF MEMBER

and parent/legal guardian will complete, sign, and date an admission agreement for each child, copying relevant information for the files when more than one child from the same family is enrolled.[CFOC3 Std. 9.4.2.3]

b. **Contents of the Agreement:**

   i.   Operating days and hours of the program

   ii.   Holiday closure dates

   iii.   Payment for services

   iv.   Drop-off and pickup procedures[CFOC3 Stds. 5.1.6.1, 6.5.2, 6.5.2.1, 9.2.4.8–9.2.4.10]

   v.   Daily sign-in and sign-out procedures[CFOC3 Std. 9.2.4.7]

   vi.   Authorized individuals for pickup of children and contact information[CFOC3 Stds. 9.2.4.8, 9.2.4.9]

   vii.   Routines to periodically test contact information (to confirm whether it is current)

   viii.   Safe passenger[CFOC3 Stds. 6.5.2.2, 6.5.2.3] and pedestrian[CFOC3 Stds. 5.1.6.1, 6.5.2.3] practices

ix.   Nonattendance and late pickup arrangements

x.   Family access to the site (whenever the child is there)[CFOC3 Std. 2.1.1.5]

xi.   Requirement for exchange of information[CFOC3 Std. 9.2.1.4]

xii. Payment of fees/deposits/refunds/late fees

xiii. Content of records[CFOC3 Std. 9.4.2.1]

xiv. Confidentiality and release of information[CFOC3 Stds. 9.4.1.3, 9.4.2.8]

xv.   Policies for health and safety[CFOC3 Std. 9.2.1.2]

xvi. Expectations for the family to provide information about the child's health and behavior (preenrollment[CFOC3 Std. 9.4.2.2] with updates whenever a change occurs[CFOC3 Std. 2.3.3.1])

xvii. Opportunities/requirements for family involvement in program activities

xviii. Primary staff member for each child (the staff member who will be the primary contact for information about the child and the specific individual[s] who will provide most of the child's care[CFOC3 Stds. 2.1.2.1, 2.1.3.1]) (See Appendix A: Child Care Admission Agreement.)

B. Enrollment (Orientation and Completion of Required Tasks Before Attendance)

1. Orientation: Prior to the child's attendance,

_____

TITLE/NAME OF STAFF MEMBER

will arrange a visit to the facility by the parent/legal guardian and child to acquaint them with the environment, staff members, program schedule, and curriculum related to the child's care. During this visit, the parent/legal guardian will have an opportunity to observe care routines, the child care group, and the teachers/caregivers who will interact with the child. Staff members will complete any special training required to care for the child before the child is allowed to enroll. Each child will spend at least

_____

MINIMUM NUMBER AND LENGTH OF VISITS

at the program with a family member before remaining in the program without a family member present. The required forms will be checked to be sure necessary information is on file prior to attendance of the child without a family member present.

2. Forms, Confidentiality, and Required Information: The parent/legal guardian will complete the following forms and submit them to

_____

TITLE/NAME OF STAFF MEMBER

prior to the child's first day of attendance. Program staff members will return any incomplete forms to the parent/legal guardian for completion prior to the child's first day of attendance and at any time during the child's enrollment and attendance when information that the facility requires needs updating.

Information concerning the child will not be made available to anyone, by any means, other than as described in this paragraph, without the expressed written consent of the parent/legal guardian.[CFOC3 Std. 9.4.1.3] Parents/legal guardians will be informed that the information will be shared with the child's teacher/caregiver, other staff members who are involved in caring for the child, consultants, and accreditation or regulation inspectors only as required to meet the needs of the child or certification of the program's operation. Except for unannounced inspections, the parent/legal guardian will be given the name(s) of the individual(s) who will be given access and the reason for giving access to confidential information.

a. **Application for Child Care Services/Enrollment Information:** Name, address, date of birth of the child; attendance date; and names, home and work addresses, all phone numbers that might be used (eg, home, cell, work), and e-mail addresses to enable contact with parents/legal guardians. Families will provide this same contact information for at least 2 additional individuals who will provide backup at any time the parents/legal guardians cannot be reached. (See Appendix B: Application for Child Care Services/ Enrollment Information.)

b. **Child Health Assessment:** Documentation of performance and findings of a checkup that includes all preventive health services, including oral health services, that the child needs according to current recommendations of the American Academy of Pediatrics. Documentation must be signed and dated by the child's physician, licensed pediatric or family nurse practitioner, or family practice physician. The information on the submitted form must be updated, initialed, and dated at each subsequent age-appropriate health assessment, or a new form must be completed, signed, and dated. Information generated by a health care professional's electronic medical record system is acceptable as long as it provides the required information. (See appendixes C: Child Health Assessment and D: Recommendations for Preventive Pediatric Health Care.)[CFOC3 Std. 9.4.2.4]

If on review of a child's health record it is determined that a nationally recommended preventive health service (eg, vision, hearing, dental examination, immunization) has not been performed,

_____

TITLE/NAME OF STAFF MEMBER

will notify the parent/legal guardian that the program requires that the health service is performed before attendance can begin or the child can continue to receive care in the program.

_____

TITLE/NAME OF STAFF MEMBER

will provide health care referrals when requested or needed. The parent/legal guardian must obtain the required health services within 6 weeks

_____

CHANGE TIME TO A PERIOD BASED ON STATE REQUIREMENTS OR PROGRAM REQUIREMENTS IF DIFFERENT

of being notified that the health service record is not up to date before the child's eligibility for enrollment is withdrawn or the child is excluded if already attending the program. If the parent/legal guardian chooses to refuse or delay the child's receipt of nationally recommended vaccines, our program _____ allow the child to receive care at our facility.

WILL/WILL NOT

If the facility accepts children whose parents refuse vaccines, add: "Our program will review, be sure parents understand, and require parents to sign and date the Refusal to Vaccinate form" and/or waivers as required by state law.

Under-immunized children may be excluded if an outbreak of a vaccine-preventable disease occurs. (See Appendix E: Refusal to Vaccinate.)

c. **Child Care Program Emergency Information:** Completed and signed by a parent/legal guardian for each child enrolled. Staff members must provide emergency information for themselves as well. Parents/legal guardians and staff members will include home, work and cell phone numbers, and name and address of the home and workplace for individuals who are their emergency contacts, and update this form quarterly and whenever information changes.*CFOC3 Std. 9.4.2.2* (See Appendix F: Staff and Child Emergency Contact and Child Pickup Information.)

d. **Special Care Plan:** When a child has a special health care need, developmental or behavioral concern, or a disability, the parent/legal guardian must inform the facility staff about this condition or concern and work with the child's specialist or health care professional(s) to complete a special care plan for that child. (See appendixes G: Special Care Plan Forms and H: How to Use Special Care Plans.) For children with special health care needs, the parent/legal guardian will have the child's health care professional complete the nationally recognized Emergency Information Form for Children With Special Needs. (See Appendix I: Emergency Information Form for Children With Special Needs.) At each health care visit, the parent/legal guardian will ask the health care professional to update information on this form and initial and date the update. To comply with the federal Health Insurance Portability and Accountability Act of 1996 regulations, the child's health care professional may require that the parent/legal guardian sign a separate form giving permission to release confidential information to the child care program. Such consent will be required if the program requires clarification from the child's health care professional of any health concerns staff members have about the child. If the program needs such information,

_____

TITLE/NAME OF STAFF MEMBER

will ask the parent/legal guardian to authorize release of information to and from providers of special services for the child to enable coordination among all services involved with the child. (See Appendix J: Authorization for Release of Information.)

e. **Consent for Child Care Program Special Activities:** For field trips and special events involving a change from the usual arrangements for child care, a special consent form must be completed by a parent/legal guardian. (See Appendix K: Consent for Child Care Program Special Activities.)

C. Attendance, Daily Record Keeping/Daily Health Checks

1. **Daily Forms:** For each child, a family member and staff member will collaborate to complete 2 forms daily.

    a. **Family-Teacher/Caregiver Information Exchange:** On daily arrival at the program site, the child's teacher/caregiver will talk with the family member and child, observe each child for signs of illness/injury that could affect the child's ability to participate in the day's activities, and with the family member, document the information. The teacher/caregiver may update the information documentation if the status of the child changes during the day. (See appendixes L: Family/Teacher–Caregiver Information Exchange Form and M: Instructions for Daily Health Check.)

    b. **Enrollment/Attendance/Symptom (E/A/S) Record:** The

_____

TITLE/NAME OF STAFF AND/OR FAMILY MEMBER

will complete the daily E/A/S record to log attendance, noting any symptom of illness/injury the child is known to have. The program will keep the written record of illness findings from these daily checks for at least 3 months and review them at least monthly to help identify outbreaks and patterns of illness for individual children and within groups of children. The E/A/S records will be reviewed by

---
TITLE/NAME OF STAFF MEMBER

to identify patterns of illness. (See Appendix N: Enrollment/Attendance/Symptom Record.)

2. **Transition to Other Programs** (See also Section 3.E: Transitions): To aid in the transition process from the facility to another school or program,

---
TITLE/NAME OF STAFF MEMBER

will inform parents/legal guardians about the availability of a summary of the child's records, needs, and special characteristics for their use. If parents/legal guardians provide written consent for sharing such information, the

---
TITLE/NAME OF STAFF MEMBER

will prepare and provide a written or verbal summary to the new source of service.[CFOC3 Std. 9.2.2.1]

3. **Termination of Enrollment:** If the parent/legal guardian terminates the child's enrollment,

---
TITLE/NAME OF STAFF MEMBER

will suggest an approach to provide a comfortable transition for the child. Refund of payments for services will be limited to _____
TIME AND AMOUNT OF ALLOWABLE REFUND.

In the event of noncompliance with the conditions described in the admission agreement and policies that the parent/legal guardian reviewed, accepted, and signed,

---
TITLE/NAME OF STAFF MEMBER

will meet with the parent/legal guardian to make a plan for corrective action that specifies the expected action and the period after which termination will occur for continued noncompliance. Program staff members will offer support to the family to achieve compliance and provide a grievance procedure that the parent/legal guardian can use. If the corrective action plan is not successful, unless the grievance procedure results in an alternative approach, termination of services will occur.

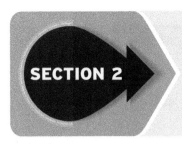

Supervision and Provision of Social-Emotional Supportive Care

Rationale

A flexible curriculum, sufficient staffing, and small group size enable verbal interaction, developmentally appropriate nurturance, and teacher/caregiver-directed and child-initiated activities. The approach reinforces children's accomplishments and promotes their continuing healthy social-emotional, cognitive, motor, and language development while keeping them safe.$^{CFOC3 \ Std. \ 1.1.1}$ Consultants can provide expertise that child care programs need. They observe, advise, provide professional development (instruct and train), refer to community resources, and provide technical assistance for program staff. Research shows that an ongoing relationship that includes periodic visits and as-needed access by a child care health consultant (CCHC) improves the quality of program performance. An early childhood education consultant who makes periodic visits can objectively assess a program and supplement the staff's knowledge of innovative ways to implement strategies to foster age-appropriate development and successfully include children with unique needs and behavioral concerns. Visits to programs that serve infants and toddlers should occur at least monthly. Visits for those that serve children 3 to 5 years of age should be at least quarterly and for school-age programs at least twice a year. Family child care homes should strive to arrange for the same frequency of CCHC visits depending on the age groups they serve.$^{CFOC3 \ Std. \ 1.6.0.2}$ Early childhood mental health consultants (ECMHCs) can suggest measures that help children who seem to be having difficulty with emotional, social, and behavioral regulation. Collaboration of these consultants with one another and with staff members and families supports children's health, learning, school readiness, and mental health. Also, it increases the ability of staff members to cope with recurring situations and reduces the stress of striving for quality care.$^{CFOC3 \ Stds. \ 1.6.0.1, \ 1.6.0.2, \ 1.6.0.3}$

Required Action/Who Is Responsible/How Communicated

A. Child:Staff Ratios, Group Size, and Staff Qualifications

1. **Overall Supervision Requirements:** Each child is always supervised by a qualified teacher/caregiver while attending the program. At least 2 staff members are always available if more than 6 children are in care. Ratios, group size, and qualifications of teacher/caregiver meet the national best practice standards.$^{CFOC3 \ Stds. \ 1.1, \ 1.2, \ 1.3, \ 1.4.4, \ 3.6.2.3, \ 3.6.2.5, \ 4.4, \ 6.5}$ Child:staff ratios and group sizes always meet or are better than the requirements of our state, territory, or tribal regulations.

2. **Supervision During Nap Time:** During nap time for children aged 31 months and older, at least one adult is physically present in the same room as the children and maximum group size is maintained. In the event that one or more children in this age group are not sleeping, such children are not made to lie down. Instead, that child or those children will move to another area to do a quiet activity with appropriate supervision. Other adults must stay on the same floor. They will immediately assist the staff member supervising sleeping children if there is an emergency during nap time. The teacher/caregiver who is in the same room with the children must be able to summon these adults without leaving the children.

3. **Ratios for Specific Activities:** This program maintains nationally specified ratios for transportation,$^{CFOC3 \ Std. \ 1.1.1.4}$ water play,$^{CFOC3 \ Std. \ 1.1.1.5}$ and inclusion of children with special needs.$^{CFOC3 \ Std. \ 1.1.1.3}$ The ratios our facility uses for daily classroom/group activities are listed in Table 2.1 for centers and Table 2.2 for large family child care homes.$^{CFOC3 \ Std. \ 1.1.1}$

Table 2.1. Child:Staff Ratios for Child Care Centers^{CFOC3 Std. 1.1.1.2}

Age	Maximum Child:Staff Ratio	Maximum Group Size
≤12-month-olds	3:1	6
13- to 35-month-olds	4:1	8
3-year-olds	7:1	14
4-year-olds	8:1	16
5-year-olds	8:1	16
6- to 8-year-olds	10:1	20
9- to 12-year-olds	12:1	24

Reprinted from American Academy of Pediatrics, American Public Health Association, National Resource Center for Health and Safety in Child Care and Early Education Programs. *Caring for Our Children: National Health and Safety Performance Standards: Guidelines for Early Care and Education Programs.* 3rd ed. Elk Grove Village, IL: American Academy of Pediatrics; 2011.

During nap time for children aged 31 months and older, at least one adult should be physically present in the same room as the children and maximum group size must be maintained. Children older than 31 months can usually be organized to nap on a schedule, but infants and toddlers as individuals are more likely to nap on different schedules. In the event even one child is not sleeping, the child should be moved to another activity where appropriate supervision is provided.

If there is an emergency during nap time, other adults should be on the same floor and should immediately assist the staff supervising sleeping children. The teacher/caregiver who is in the same room with the children should be able to summon these adults without leaving the children.

When there are mixed-age groups in the same room, the child:staff ratio and group size should be consistent with the age of most of the children. When infants or toddlers are in the mixed-age group, the child:staff ratio and group size for infants and toddlers should be maintained. In large family child care homes with 2 or more teachers/caregivers caring for no more than 12 children, no more than 3 children younger than 2 years should be in care.

Children with special health care needs or who require more attention because of certain disabilities may require additional staff on-site, depending on their special needs and the extent of their disabilities.

At least one adult who has satisfactorily completed a course in pediatric first aid, including cardiopulmonary resuscitation (CPR) skills, within the past 3 years should be part of the ratio at all times.

Table 2.2. Child:Staff Ratios for Large Family Child Care (Group) Homes^{CFOC3 Std. 1.1.1.2}

Age	Maximum Child:Staff Ratio	Maximum Group Size
≤12-month-olds	2:1	6
13- to 23-month-olds	2:1	8
24- to 35-month-olds	3:1	12
3-year-olds	7:1	12
4- to 5-year-olds	8:1	12
6- to 8-year-olds	10:1	12
9- to 12-year-olds	12:1	12

Reprinted from American Academy of Pediatrics, American Public Health Association, National Resource Center for Health and Safety in Child Care and Early Education Programs. *Caring for Our Children: National Health and Safety Performance Standards: Guidelines for Early Care and Education Programs.* 3rd ed. Elk Grove Village, IL: American Academy of Pediatrics; 2011.

During nap time for children younger than 30 months, the child:staff ratio must be maintained at all times regardless of how many children are sleeping. They must also be maintained even during the adult's break time so that ratios are not relaxed.

B. Supervision of Children

1. **Line of Sight and Hearing:** Teachers/caregivers directly supervise infant, toddler, and preschool children by line of sight and hearing at all times, even when the children are sleeping. *Line of sight* means that the teacher/caregiver can see the children without more than a turn or tilt of the head.[CFOC3 Std. 2.2.0.1]

2. **Counting Children:** Teachers/caregivers regularly count children on a scheduled basis, at every transition, and whenever the group is leaving one area and arriving at another to confirm the safe whereabouts of every child at all times. A system to remind staff members to count at prescribed intervals, such as a reminder tone that sounds every 10 to 15 minutes, is used to help teachers/caregivers remember to count.

_____
TITLE/NAME OF STAFF MEMBER

assigns and reassigns counting responsibility to make sure that each child remains under the direct supervision of and is counted by a specified teacher/caregiver.

3. **Evaluation and Removal of Environmental Barriers to Supervision:**

_____
TITLE/NAME OF STAFF MEMBER

observes group activities

_____ to assess the environment for opportunities to improve visibility and hearing of
FREQUENCY
child activities. Visibility may be improved through the use of devices such as convex mirrors or screens linked with cameras mounted in locations that are sometimes hard to view from all areas being used by the group.

4. **Limits on Independence and Privacy:** School-aged children may be out of sight briefly, ie, no more than 5 minutes, to use the toilet, complete an errand within the building, go to a library area of the building to get a book, or carry out a similar age-appropriate brief independent activity as long as the child can be heard by a teacher/caregiver (eg, while using the toilet) or, if the child is going to a different part of the facility, a responsible adult expects the arrival of the child in a timely fashion.

   A teacher/caregiver is always on the same floor level as the children. The school-aged child's teacher/caregiver should be close by and listening carefully to be sure all children are safe and engaged in appropriate activities. Children are never outdoors or inside by themselves. Older preschool- and school-aged children who are able to use the toilet independently are allowed privacy for toileting but are within hearing of a supervising teacher/caregiver. The teacher/caregiver makes sure that children use the toilet and hand-washing facilities as intended.[CFOC3 Std. 2.2.0.1]

5. **Community Outreach and Involvement for School-aged Children:** School-aged children have opportunities to participate in community outreach and involvement such as field trips and community improvement activities as approved by their parent/legal guardian and teacher/caregiver.[CFOC3 Std. 2.1.4.5] School-aged children may, with written approval of a parent/guardian and teacher/caregiver, participate in activities off the premises that are not operated by the program, but the facility is not to be responsible for the child during the off-premises activity.[CFOC3 Std. 2.2.0.1]

6. **Active Supervision Measures:** All teachers/caregivers practice active supervision,$^{CFOC3\ Std.\ 2.2.0.1}$ including the following measures recommended by the Head Start Early Childhood Knowledge & Learning Center[1]:

   a. **Focused Attention and Observation of Children:** At all times, including while interacting with individual children—watching, counting, and listening for sounds or the absence of sounds that raise concern. Teachers/caregivers limit adult-adult socializing to break times or when they have made arrangements to delegate supervision of children to another teacher/caregiver. They do not talk on cell phones or use text messages or other forms of social media while supervising children, except to summon help in an emergency.

   b. **Knowing Each Child:** Teachers/caregivers strive to know each child's abilities, anticipating challenges that might lead to harmful or undesirable behavior.

   c. **Setting Up the Environment:** All areas are easy to view and free of distracting sounds that hinder hearing what children are doing. Spaces are free of clutter and trip hazards. They are organized for safe storage that allows only appropriate access to materials without risking a fall or having materials fall. There are clear and simple safety rules that are consistently reinforced.

   d. **Choosing Strategic Positions:** Teachers/caregivers position themselves where they can observe all the children and scan play activities in the entire area while remaining directly responsible for close supervision of those specifically/individually assigned to them.

   e. **Scanning for Hazards:** Each teacher/caregiver remains aware of and scans the indoor and outdoor environments and activities for potential safety hazards. (See Appendix O: Daily and Monthly Playground Inspection and Maintenance.)

   f. **Focusing on the Positive:** Teachers/caregivers explain and model for children what is safe for the child and other children (eg, teaching children the appropriate and safe use of each piece of equipment such as using a slide correctly—feet first only—and explaining why climbing up a slide can cause injury and that going down the slide headfirst can result in a head injury).

   g. **Photo Identification and Correct Spelling of Children's Legal First and Last Names as Well as Nicknames:** Teachers/caregivers not only know the number of children in the group but also the correctly spelled legal first and last names and nicknames of all children for whom the teacher/caregiver is responsible. This is especially important when a child in the group has a special need, when there are many new children in the group, when there is a substitute teacher/caregiver, or at early and late points in the day when the teacher/caregiver may not know the children as well as those who care for them at other times of the day. Each group has a current photo and name display to positively identify each child in the group. Only the name and face of the child should be in the display. Other information should be kept confidential, except that parents/legal guardians should authorize display of essential information to care for a child's special need such as a food allergy.

7. **Mixed-Age Groups:** When there are mixed-age groups in the same room, the child:staff ratio and group size is consistent with the age of the majority of children unless there are infants or toddlers in the mixed-age group. When infants or toddlers are in the group, the child:staff ratio and group size for infants and toddlers is maintained. When children who have special needs are in the group, the facility determines if additional staff members must be present to provide quality child care for all children in the group.$^{CFOC3\ Std.\ 1.1.1.3}$

8. **Substitutes and Volunteers:** A substitute may be employed or a volunteer assigned so that the required child:staff ratios are maintained at all times. Substitutes and volunteers must be at least 18 years of age and have the same qualifications for their roles, preservice clearances and training, and must review, sign, and date acknowledgment of program policies and procedures as required of the staff members who regularly work in the facility. Any substitute without a teacher/caregiver license, certificate, or education and experience qualifications required of the regular teacher/caregiver works under direct supervision of a person with the recommended credentials and is not left alone with a group of children at any time. A substitute who is regularly employed as a teacher/caregiver by the facility and who is well-known by the children in the group is considered a staff member and may function in the same way as the teacher/caregiver for whom the substitution is being made.$^{CFOC3\ Std.\ 1.5.0.1}$

C. Supervision of Active (Large-Muscle) Play

1. **Supervised Play:** Teachers/caregivers use the measures described in Section 2.B.6 for active supervision of children by sight and sound during active (large-muscle) play in indoor and outdoor spaces. High-risk play areas (ie, climbers, slides, swings, and water play) receive the most staff attention. All children using playground or indoor play equipment are directly supervised and monitored closely by teachers/caregivers. Children are not permitted to go beyond a teacher's/caregiver's ability to provide direct supervision by sight and sound. Child:staff ratios are at least as stringent as for other child care activities.

2. **Counting Children at Timed Intervals:** Every child is specifically assigned to a teacher/caregiver to be regularly counted at timed intervals of no longer than 15 minutes to confirm the child's safe whereabouts at all times during active (large-muscle) play times.

_____

TITLE/NAME OF STAFF MEMBER

prepares a written schedule to assign staff to supervise high-risk areas. (See Appendix P: Staff Assignments for Active [Large-Muscle] Play.)

D. Swimming, Wading, Gross Motor Water Play

1. **Water Activities:** When swimming, wading, or other gross motor play activities in water are part of the program, each infant or toddler has 1:1 supervision with a teacher/caregiver having a hand on the infant or toddler at all times during the activity. For preschool-aged children, the required child:staff ratio during water activities for preschoolers is 4:1, and for school-aged children, 6:1.[CFOC3 Std. 1.1.1.5]

2. **Supervision of Large-Muscle Water Play:** The supervising teacher/caregiver is not involved in any activity other than directly supervising the assigned child(ren) and must have current certification of successful completion of a course in pediatric first aid and CPR.

E. Consultants and Child Care Health Advocate[CFOC3 Stds. 1.3.2.7, 1.6]

1. **Health Consultant:** The health professional who serves as this facility's CCHC is

_____

NAME

Our CCHC visits this facility

_____

SPECIFY FREQUENCY (EG, WEEKLY, MONTHLY. SHOULD BE AT LEAST MONTHLY FOR INFANTS AND TODDLERS, QUARTERLY FOR CHILDREN 3–5 YEARS OF AGE, TWICE ANNUALLY FOR SCHOOL-AGED CHILDREN.)

in addition to being available to answer questions of staff members by phone or e-mail.

2. **Health Advocate:** This facility's child care health advocate is

_____

NAME

In addition to other roles in our program, our child care health advocate makes sure the key tasks related to health and safety are done. Our health advocate may not do all required tasks but makes sure that all are done. Our child care health advocate coordinates with our CCHC to be sure we follow best practices for health and safety.

3. **Early Childhood Mental Health Consultant:** This facility's ECMHC,

_____

NAME

comes at least quarterly to observe and advise staff members about child development and strategies to manage behavioral concerns.

4. **Early Childhood Educational Consultant:** This facility's early childhood educational consultant,

_____

NAME

comes at least semiannually to observe and advise staff members about teaching strategies and other aspects of the educational components of the program.

F. Family/Staff Communication

1. **Types of Communication:** Staff members promote communication between themselves and the families of children in the facility with short daily verbal communications, supplemented by written notes and planned (and documented) conferences with parents/legal guardians. Families are encouraged to leave/send written notes with important information so all teachers/caregivers who work with the child can share the parents' communication.[CFOC3 Std. 2.3.2.1]

2. **Frequency of Communications:** Teachers/caregivers write dated notes using forms or the facility's stationary that includes the facility's name and contact information to communicate with families of infants and toddlers _____ for infants _____, for preschool and
   FREQUENCY OF NOTE WRITING (EG, DAILY)   FREQUENCY (EG, WEEKLY)

   kindergarten children, and no less than _____ for school-aged children.
   FREQUENCY (EG, MONTHLY)

   Staff members use these notes to inform families about the child's experiences, accomplishments, behavior, sleeping, feeding, injuries, changes in health status, and other issues related to personal care such as wet diapers and bowel movements for infants and toddlers.

3. **Use of Documented Communications:** Communications/notes are recorded and collected to assess and share the child's progress with families, staff members, and any professionals involved with the child. The notes help track the course of the child's progress and may reveal any problems or patterns of behavior that cause concern.

_____

TITLE/NAME OF STAFF MEMBER

schedules a conference with the parent/legal guardian any time there is a concern and no less than every 6 months for children younger than 6 years and annually for older children. Staff members do not use e-mail communications to send confidential information related to medical, behavioral, or other personal details that could be intercepted.

Reference

1.   Office of Head Start. Active Supervision: A Referenced Fact Sheet From the Head Start National Center on Health. Washington, DC: Office of Head Start; 2013

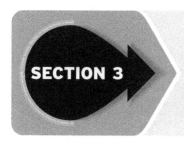

Planned Program, Teaching, and Guidance

Rationale

A planned program, curriculum, and effective teaching practices enable parents and staff members to know what to expect and to work cooperatively. Play is the foundation of the planned curriculum. Learning occurs best in situations that accept differences among individuals and reinforces areas of strength while strengthening areas of weakness. Children thrive when their teachers/caregivers have trusting, respectful, consistent, affectionate relationships with them in an environment that provides developmentally appropriate opportunities for learning. These opportunities include exploration, manipulation of objects and ideas, and an abundance of meaningful self-initiated experiences. Cognitive, physical, social-emotional, and communication skills are interdependent.

Health and safety affect all types of learning and are best addressed as integrated components of all aspects of child care. Children learn and demonstrate expected behavior when their teachers/caregivers are supportive and caring role models. The meaning of discipline is teaching, not punishment. The facility's clearly stated principles guide the program and help achieve consensus about how and what staff members include in activities and approaches they use. A written description of the planned program of daily activities allows staff members and parents/guardians to have a common understanding and compare the program's actual performance with the stated intent. Planning for indoor and outdoor programming for children also provides a tool for staff orientation. Used as a reference point for evaluation of staff member performance, a written statement of principles and description of the planned daily program provide a rational basis for staff members to receive professional development.[CFOC3 Stds. 2.1.1–2.1.4]

Required Action/Who Is Responsible/How Communicated

A. Philosophy of Teaching, Guidance, and Behavior Management

Teachers/caregivers will competently explain to families and coworkers the philosophy of the program as expressed in written principles. The explanation includes how the principles are reflected in the purpose and specific activities of the planned daily program and curriculum the teachers/caregivers are implementing.

_____

TITLE/NAME OF STAFF MEMBER

uses the program's statement of principles, planned daily program, and curriculum as the basis of observations, evaluations, and professional development to improve staff performance.

B. Permissible Methods for Teaching, Behavior Management, and Discipline*CFOC3* Stds. 2.2.0.6–2.2.0.10

1. **Teacher/Caregiver Interactions With Children:** Teachers/caregivers support social and emotional learning by talking and listening to the child and playing with and responding to the child's needs. They lead, using positive guidance and redirection, planning ahead to prevent problems, encouraging appropriate behavior, using consistent clear rules, and whenever possible, involving in problem solving to foster the child's own ability to become self-regulated. If the child understands words, logical (disciplinary) consequences are explained simply to the child before misbehavior occurs and at the time of any disciplinary action. Teachers/ caregivers encourage children to respect other people, be fair, respect property, and learn to be responsible for their actions.

2. **Coordinated Approach to Discipline:** Program staff members work with families and everyone else who cares for the child to use the following approaches for discipline:

   a. **Ensure Active Participation of Each Child:** Encourage desired behavior by providing engaging materials based on children's interests, ensuring that the learning environment promotes active participation of each child.

   b. **Teach Social Competence:** Help children learn what to expect in the child care environment and how to promote positive interactions and engagement with others.

   c. **Children Experience Predictable Routines:** Provide a predictable daily schedule with routines, activities, reminders, and transitions to foster the desired behaviors.

   d. **Match Expectations of Behavior to the Child's Development:** By understanding what abilities the child has acquired and is expected to do as a next step in development, adults can facilitate smooth and steady progress in self-mastery and independent pro-social behaviors (eg, toddlers want to demonstrate their independence and often say "no" to a yes-or-no choice but happily choose between 2 equally acceptable alternatives).

   e. **Simple Rules:** Establish, teach, and support learning of simple rules expressed as what to do, rather than what not to do.

   f. **Praise:** Positively describe the desired behavior (eg, "You did a nice job putting your toy away," rather than global, nonspecific praise such as "Good girl" or "Nice job").

   g. **Model Desired Behavior:** Model and demonstrate to help children understand positive alternative behaviors as the first approach to correcting a behavior that is not acceptable (eg, lower your voice when the child is yelling).

   h. **Planned Ignoring and Redirecting:** Suggest another activity unless the behavior is too disruptive and unsafe to be ignored.

   i. **Individualize Discipline:** Adjust the approach to the temperament and needs of the child, anticipating and preventing situations that are likely to evoke undesirable behavior.

   j. **Limit Use of Time-out:** Select one persistent unacceptable behavior that will predictably result in a time-out experience. Use this method only for children who are older than 2 years, and then only to interrupt the unacceptable behavior for a short period, usually no more than 1 minute per year of age. End the period of time-out with a positive statement about the child's ability to do what is expected.

3. **Handling Physical Aggression and Other Behaviors of Concern:** Teachers/caregivers intervene immediately when a child becomes physically aggressive to protect all of the children and encourage more acceptable behavior.*CFOC3* Std. 2.2.0.6 For acts of aggression and fighting (eg, biting, hitting), the teacher/ caregiver tells the child clearly that the aggressive behavior is not allowed (eg, "No biting"; "No hitting"). The teacher/caregiver tells verbal children what is appropriate (eg, "We bite food"; "We use words to say 'I am angry'").*CFOC3* Std. 2.2.0.7 In addition, the teacher/caregiver may separate the children involved, immediately

comfort and care for any injury to the victim of the aggressor, and notify parents/legal guardians of the children involved in the incident about what happened and how the situation was resolved. The families of the children need to understand if the child relates to the experience during time at home. However, families are discouraged from disciplining their children additionally for an incident unless it is part of a coordinated plan made with the child's teacher/caregiver. Although the children may say who was involved, teachers/caregivers will not identify the victim to the family of the aggressor or the aggressor to the family of the victim.

a. **Assessment:**

_____

TITLE/NAME OF STAFF MEMBER

assesses the adequacy of teacher/caregiver supervision, appropriateness of facility activities, possible disruptive factors in the child's life (eg, parental stress, change in household composition, illness), and what the administrative corrective action would be if the aggressive behavior continues.

b. **Mental Health Consultation:**

_____

TITLE/NAME OF STAFF MEMBER

arranges quarterly visits by an early childhood mental health consultant to observe teacher/caregiver interactions with the child and advise staff members about approaches to manage behaviors that are causing concern.[CFOC3 Std. 1.6.0.3] This program explicitly prohibits corporal punishment, psychological abuse, humiliation, abusive language, binding or tying to restrict movement, restriction of access to large-motor physical activities, and withdrawal or forcing of food and other basic needs.[CFOC3 Std. 2.2.0.9] Before they are hired, all teachers/caregivers sign an agreement to implement the facility's discipline policies that includes the consequence for staff members who do not follow the discipline policies. If a child's behavior is unresponsive to the usually effective discipline measures described previously, the program will seek help from a qualified early childhood mental health consultant.

4. **Prohibited Behaviors:** The following behaviors are prohibited in our facility. Some may require mandatory reporting of an instance of child abuse.[CFOC3 Std. 2.2.0.9]

   a. **Use of Any Form of Corporal Punishment:** Corporal punishment means punishment inflicted directly on the body—hitting, spanking, shaking, slapping, twisting, pulling, squeezing hurtfully, demanding excessive physical exercise that most children cannot pleasurably do, forced rest, adoption of bizarre positions, compelling a child to eat or put soap/food/spices/foreign substances in the child's mouth, exposing a child to extreme temperatures without proper clothing or protection, isolating a child in an adjacent room/hallway/closet/dark area/play area/any area where the child is not seen and supervised, trying to restrict movement by binding or strapping into a seat except a car seat when traveling in a vehicle, taping, using or withholding food as punishment or reward, or taking away physical activity/outdoor time as punishment.

   b. **Coercive Toilet Learning:** Toilet learning/training methods that punish, demean, or humiliate a child.

   c. **Emotional Abuse:** Any form of emotional abuse, including rejecting, terrorizing, extended ignoring, isolating, or corrupting a child.

   d. **Other Abuse or Maltreatment:** Any abuse or maltreatment of a child, including exposure of any child to pornographic material of any nature via electronic devices or printed material, as an incident of discipline, or as any other inappropriate practice.

   e. **Abusive Language:** Abusive, profane, or sarcastic language or verbal abuse, threats, or derogatory remarks about the child or child's family.

   f. **Humiliation or Threats:** Any form of public or private humiliation, including threats of physical punishment.

C. Developmentally Appropriate Care

1. **Routines for All Age Groups:** During daily routines (eg, feeding, play, diapering, hand washing, active play indoors and outdoors), teachers/caregivers comfort children, play and socially interact with them verbally, use positive facial expressions and a pleasant tone of voice and actions, and integrate required health and safety practices. At the time transitions occur for care of the child from the family to a staff member and back again, program staff members and families will use a consistent method to receive and give communication about the child's experiences and routines at home and while in the program. Communication about any unusual event or circumstance occurs promptly no matter when it occurs.

2. **Infants and Toddlers**

    a. Our facility accepts care for children when they are at least[CFOC3 Std. 1.1.2.1]

    _____

    MINIMUM AGE OF ENROLLMENT.

    b. **Separation of Age Groups:** Children in center-based care who are younger than 3 years have teachers/caregivers and receive care in rooms that they do not share concurrently with older children unless special arrangements to care for children in mixed-age groups has been made.

    c. **Primary Teacher/Caregiver Assignments:** Assignments for teachers/caregivers to specific children minimize the number of teachers/caregivers interacting with each child during a given day and reduce the risk of injury and spread of infectious diseases.[CFOC3 Stds. 2.1] Teachers/caregivers provide consistent, continuous care. No more than 5 teachers/caregivers participate in the infant's/toddler's care during a year.

    _____

    TITLE/NAME OF STAFF MEMBER

    designates one of these as the primary teacher/caregiver, the person most responsible for having a long-term, trusting relationship with the child and family, for making sure program policies are followed and communication between staff and family members occurs. Additional specialists may be involved with the child to address special needs or unique learning opportunities as long as the primary teacher/caregiver monitors and supports the child for these experiences.[CFOC3 Stds. 2.1.2]

    d. **Toilet Learning:** Toilet learning occurs when the child shows readiness for using the toilet and the family is ready to support the child's involvement in doing so. Readiness indicators include desire to perform self-body care, ability to remain dry for at least 2 hours at a time, communication skills to understand and express concepts related to toileting, ability to get onto and sit with minimal assistance on a toilet adapted for the child's size or appropriately sized, and awareness of the sensations associated with releasing urine and stool.[CFOC3 Std. 2.1.2.5]

    e. **Outdoor Time and Physical Activity for Infants and Toddlers:** Infants are taken outside 2 to 3 times per day, as tolerated, and have supervised tummy time while awake every day. Toddlers (12 months– 3 years) receive 60 to 90 minutes of outdoor play, weather permitting.[CFOC3 Std. 3.1.3.1]

3. Preschool-aged Children

a. **Primary Teacher/Caregiver Assignment:** To build long-term, trusting relationships, the program limits the number of teachers/caregivers and other adults who care for any one preschool-aged child to no more than 8 adults in a given year and no more than 3 teachers/caregivers in one day. These staff members are considered primary teachers/caregivers.

TITLE/NAME OF STAFF MEMBER

designates one of these as the person most responsible for having a long-term, trusting relationship with the child and family. This primary teacher/caregiver makes sure program policies related to the child's care are followed and that timely communications between staff and family members occur. Additional specialists may be involved with the child to address special needs or unique learning opportunities as long as the primary teacher/caregiver monitors and supports the child for these experiences.[CFOC3 Std. 2.1.3.1]

b. **Structure of the Curriculum:** Teachers/caregivers plan and provide a balance of guided and self-initiated play and learning indoors and outdoors. Children observe, explore, order and reorder, make mistakes and find solutions, and move from concrete to abstract learning.[CFOC3 Std. 2.1.3.2]

c. **Teachers/Caregivers Foster Cooperation Rather Than Competition:** The curriculum includes expressive activities such as free play, painting, drawing, storytelling, sensory activities, music, singing, dancing, and taking part in drama, all of which integrate thinking and feeling and foster socialization, conflict resolution, and language and cognitive development.[CFOC3 Std. 2.1.3.4]

d. **Language Development:** Teachers/caregivers encourage children's language development using reading, speaking and listening interactively, responding to questions about observations and feelings, storytelling, and writing.[CFOC3 Std. 2.1.3.6]

e. **Body Mastery:** To encourage body mastery, the curriculum includes learning socially acceptable self-feeding, appropriate use of the toilet, and large- and small-muscle activities.[CFOC3 Std. 2.1.3.7]

f. **Physical Activity:** Preschoolers have 90 to 120 minutes per 8-hour day of moderate to vigorous activities.[CFOC3 Std. 3.1.3.1]

g. **School-aged Children:** The program provides supervised before- and after-school and vacation time care for school-aged children. The curriculum includes physical activity, healthful nutrition, recreation, completion of schoolwork, social relationships, and use of community resources, all of which are coordinated with school and home life. Activities include free play, at least 60 minutes of indoor and outdoor physical activity, time and settings for schoolwork and recreation alone or in a group, field trips to community facilities, relationships with understanding and comforting adults, and rest.[CFOC3 Std. 2.1.4.1] Regular communications occur at least _____ among the children's schoolteachers,
FREQUENCY OF COMMUNICATIONS
parents/legal guardians, and child care program staff members.[CFOC3 Std. 2.1.4.6]

D. Required Clothing for Children and Staff Members

1. **Suitable Clothing:** Teachers/caregivers and children wear clothing that permits easy and safe movement as well as full participation in active and messy play. Children are not allowed to wear clothing that has strings or decorations that can get caught on equipment. Children and staff members must have suitable clothing at the facility for going outdoors when it is raining or snowing to allow children to use these opportunities to learn about the natural world and how to function in it.

2. **Footwear:** Footwear must be the equivalent of gym shoes that are not slippery, will not twist or come off the feet while running, and stay firmly on the feet while climbing, jumping, skipping, and crawling.[CFOC3 Std. 9.2.3.1] Footwear is not permitted that provides insufficient support for or limits active play, such as shoes with heels, flip-flops, loose boots, or dress shoes.

3. **Spare Clothing:** Staff members keep a spare set of clothing and shoes to wear in the event their clothing becomes heavily soiled or wet or is in contact with blood or other body fluids during the program day. Program staff members remove clothing or shoes that are badly soiled or damaged or that interfere with active play or comfort. Such articles are exchanged with the spare set of clothing and shoes.

E. Transitions

1. **Communications for Transitions:** Transitions at the beginning, during, and at the end of the program day are accompanied by written and verbal communication between whoever has responsibility for the care of the child and whoever is assuming responsibility from someone else. These communications involve family members and teachers/caregivers at drop-off/pickup times and other times when something of concern has occurred during the caregiving day. In addition, written documentation and verbal communication occur whenever a primary teacher/caregiver transfers caring responsibility to another staff member. Documentation of each transition includes who was involved, what was reported about the child's needs and experiences, and when the transition occurred. This documentation is kept as part of the child's record.[CFOC3 Std. 9.2.2.3]

2. **Advance Planning for Transitions:** Transitions that require advance planning include attendance at a special program while continuing to be enrolled in the child care program or leaving the child care program on a permanent basis. Collaborative planning for such transitions involves

_____

TITLE/NAME OF STAFF MEMBER

and the child's primary teacher(s)/caregiver(s), parent/legal guardian, and with consent of the parent/legal guardian, staff members from the program where the child is going.

_____

TITLE/NAME OF STAFF MEMBER

prepares a summary of the child's records and progress while in the child care program and give copies of this summary to the family and, with parent/legal guardian consent, to the staff person(s) from the other source of service. For children with special needs,

_____

TITLE/NAME OF STAFF MEMBER

organizes a joint conference that involves staff members from the child care program the child currently attends and the program where the child is going and the parents/legal guardians.[CFOC3 Std. 9.2.2.1]

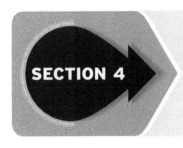

Nutrition, Food Handling, and Feeding

Rationale

Current research shows that children need a variety of nutrient-dense foods that include protein, carbohydrates, oils, vitamins, and minerals, with an amount of calories that prevents hunger, fosters healthy growth, and prevents obesity. The best first food is human milk, which is commonly called breast milk. Formula is an adequate substitute when human milk is not available. Children learn to self-feed and develop lifelong healthful habits by being introduced to developmentally appropriate solids and observing eating modeled by others. Because children pick and choose from different kinds and combinations of foods offered, healthful foods should be offered at each feeding. After 1 year of age, children need to drink water as a beverage when they have consumed the recommended amount of milk at a meal and as the between-meal beverage. Overconsumption of juice contributes to overweight/obesity, malnutrition, and dental decay. Overconsumption of milk is associated with iron deficiency anemia.[1,2]

Compliance with food service standards for food handling is essential to avoid food-borne illness and exposure of children to foods to which they are allergic. These precautions apply to ordering, receiving, storing, preparing, and serving food.[CFOC3 Chapter 4]

Required Action/Who Is Responsible/How Communicated

A. Acceptable Food and Drink

1. Staff Role

    a. **Food and Beverages Consumed by Adults in This Facility:** In the presence of children, unless there is a medical contraindication that requires otherwise, all adults drink beverages and eat fruits and vegetables and meats or meat alternatives such as beans and grains that are being served to children.

    b. **Teachers/Caregivers Provide Nutrition Education**

        i. Teachers/caregivers observe and support children's healthy eating habits and hunger and fullness cues.

        ii. All staff members make sure that the food offered to children meets the recommendations of the Institute of Medicine for the US Department of Agriculture (USDA) Child and Adult Care Food Program, which are posted on the USDA Food and Nutrition Service Web site.[3,4]

2. Beverages

a. **Water:** Clean, sanitary drinking water is available throughout the day when children are indoors or outdoors. Only cold water taps are used to draw drinking water or water for cooking. The US Environmental Protection Agency (EPA) recommends that "Anytime the water in a particular faucet has not been used for six hours or longer, 'flush' your cold-water pipes by running the water until it becomes as cold as it will get. This could take as little as five to thirty seconds if there has been recent heavy water use.… Otherwise, it could take two minutes or longer. Your water utility will inform you if longer flushing times are needed to respond to local conditions."[5]

_____
TITLE/NAME OF STAFF MEMBER

contacted the local health department on _____ to be sure the program's
                                          DATE

source of drinking water is free of lead, parasites, bacteria, and other contaminants and determined that
the tap water at this facility _____ fluoridated. (If the facility uses well water,
                                IS/IS NOT

the alternate policy is: The well that serves our facility is checked for chemical and bacterial contamination at least annually.)

Prior to 12 months of age, infants are offered their mother's breast milk or formula, not water, for extra hydration on hot days, unless otherwise directed by the child's health care professional in writing. On hot days or when they have been physically active, all children older than 12 months are offered water to drink. All children older than 12 months are offered water for oral hygiene whenever they do not brush their teeth after a snack or meal. Water is offered in a cup or, if the child can drink without touching the water outlet, from a drinking fountain. Water is available at meals and snacks but is not substituted for milk when milk is a required food component unless recommended by the child's health care professional.$^{CFOC3\ Std.\ 4.2.0.6}$

b. **Milk:** Children younger than 12 months do not receive cow's milk unless the child's health care professional gives a written exception and direction to do so. Between 12 and 24 months of age, children who do not drink their mother's breast milk or prescribed formula can have whole pasteurized milk or reduced-fat (2%) pasteurized milk as recommended by the child's health care professional. Children 2 years and older are served nonfat (skim) or low-fat (1%) pasteurized milk.$^{CFOC3\ Std.\ 4.3.1.7}$ Unpasteurized (raw) milk is not served.

c. **Allowable Beverages:** Children younger than 12 months do not receive juice. Children between 1 and 6 years of age receive no more than a total of 4 to 6 ounces of 100% juice per day, including juice given at home. Children who are 7 to 12 years of age receive no more than a total of 8 to 12 ounces of juice per day, including any juice consumed at home. During functions or meetings attended only by adults, water, tea, coffee, or milk is served.$^{CFOC3\ Std.\ 4.2.0.7}$

d. **Use of Bottles or Spill-resistant Cups:** Adults and children may not carry around beverages in a cup, can, bottle, or spill-resistant cup. Children do not receive any food or drink in a bottle other than human milk or iron-fortified infant formula unless the child's health care professional gives a written direction to do so.

3. Fruits and Vegetables

a. **Encouragement of Tasting:** Staff members gently encourage children to try developmentally appropriate servings of fruits and vegetables and offer positive reinforcement when a child does so.

b. **Fruits and Vegetables Instead of Sweets:** During celebrations and holiday parties, children are offered developmentally appropriate servings of fruits and vegetables rather than foods with a high percentage of sugars, salts, or fats. See the approved list of age-appropriate foods for celebrations available from

_____

TITLE/NAME OF STAFF MEMBER.

c. **Fruits and Vegetables in Foods Brought From Home:** Families are expected to include fruits and vegetables in packed lunches or any other food brought from home.

_____

TITLE/NAME OF STAFF MEMBER

will provide examples and resources to help families provide a variety of fruits and vegetables.

d. **Washing All Fruits and Vegetables:** The first step in preparation of all fruits and vegetables is cleaning them with a vegetable brush and water.

4. Meat and Meat Alternatives:
For packed meals from home, families are expected to provide developmentally appropriate servings of protein such as lean meat, skinless poultry, fish, cooked beans or peas, nut butters, eggs, yogurt, or cheese. Commercial prepackaged lunches or baked pre-fried or high-fat meats such as chicken nuggets and hot dogs are not permitted. See _____ for the approved

TITLE/NAME OF STAFF MEMBER

list of age-appropriate meat and meat alternatives.

5. Grain and Bread:
High-fat products (containing >35% of calories from fat) and high-sugar products (containing >35% of calories from sugar) are not permitted. A list of approved age-appropriate grain foods for parties and celebrations that meet the guidelines is available from

_____

TITLE/NAME OF STAFF MEMBER.

Breads, pastas, and grains are made from whole grains when possible. Whole grain cereals are served and contain no more than 6 grams of sugar per serving. High-sugar, high-sodium, or high-fat snack items are not served.

B. Food Brought From Home _CFOC3_ Stds. 4.6.0.1, 4.6.0.2

1. Informing Families About Acceptable Foods:

_____

TITLE/NAME OF STAFF MEMBER

informs parents or legal guardians about the food service plan of the facility and suggest ways to coordinate with this plan. An approved list of age-appropriate foods that can be brought from home is available from

_____

TITLE/NAME OF STAFF MEMBER.

This list matches the recommendations of the Institute of Medicine for the USDA Child and Adult Care Food Program (See Section 4.A.1.b.ii).

2. **Supplementation of Food Brought From Home:** The program supplements a child's home-provided meal if the nutritional content appears to be inadequate.

_____

TITLE/NAME OF STAFF MEMBER

informs the parent or legal guardian if food brought from home is being supplemented on a regular basis. Teachers/caregivers check for food allergies before providing any supplemental food.

3. **Situations When Food May Be Brought From Home**

   a. **For Special Occasions:** All special event celebration plans require prior approval from

   _____

   TITLE/NAME OF STAFF MEMBER

   including approval of the activities, materials, and any food involved. Staff members encourage parents to celebrate their child's birthday or other special occasions with an alternative to food, such as sharing favorite stories, music, dancing, games, crafts, or other activities. What is important to children is that their families planned something special. Using food as the focus of celebrations is discouraged. If perishable food is brought from home to be shared with other children, it must be store bought, in its original package, and in a quantity sufficient for all of the children. Children may not share food provided by the child's family unless the food is intended for sharing with all of the children.

   b. **Meals (Lunch, Snack):** Families may provide food for their child described in a written agreement signed and dated by the parent/legal guardian and

   _____

   TITLE/NAME OF STAFF MEMBER.

   These foods include protein such as lean meat, skinless poultry, fish, cooked beans or peas, nut butters, eggs, yogurt, or cheese; fruit and vegetables; and grain products such as cereals, crackers, breads, pastas, brown rice, and other whole grains.

   c. **Nutrient Requirements for Foods:** This facility does not permit commercially prepackaged lunches that do not meet the requirements of the USDA Child and Adult Care Food Program or baked pre-fried or high-fat meats such as chicken nuggets and hot dogs; high-fat products (containing >35% of calories from fat); and high-sugar products (containing >35% of calories from sugar). Intake of sodium is limited by not adding salt to prepared foods and selecting foods that are low in sodium content.[6,7]

4. **Preparation, Transport, and Safe Food Temperatures:** Lunch and snack foods brought from home must be prepared and transported in a sanitary fashion, including maintenance of safe food temperatures for perishable items.

_____

TITLE/NAME OF STAFF MEMBER

checks foods brought from home when the food arrives at the facility. Perishable foods are checked with a thermometer if they do not seem cold or hot enough on arrival. Food that is not at a safe temperature when it arrives is discarded. Checking of food brought from home includes a determination of food safety and storage requirements for the food when it arrives at the facility. Perishable foods that require refrigeration are kept cold, at or below 41°F, and perishable hot foods are kept hot, at or above 135°F, until served, when they are allowed to cool to 110°F so they will not cause burns. Foods must be eaten or discarded within 2 hours of being out of the safe temperatures for holding food.[CFOC3 Stds. 4.8.0.6, 4.10.0.2] Families should label food brought from home with the child's full name, date, type of food, and any need for temperature control.

5. **Leftovers:** Staff members discard any leftover food. The only food that staff members may return to the family is unopened commercially wrapped food that does not require refrigeration or holding at a hot temperature.

C. Food Prepared at or for the Facility and Served at the Facility

1. Food and Nutrition Service Plan:

_____

TITLE/NAME OF STAFF MEMBER

designates responsible individuals and drafts plans related to food and nutrition service in consultation with a nutritionist/registered dietitian with pediatric expertise.

a. **Content of Food Service Plan:** The following items are addressed in the plans monitored by

_____

TITLE/NAME OF STAFF MEMBER

and kept for reference and review[CFOC3 Stds. 4.2.0.1, 9.2.3.11] in

_____

LOCATION OF PLANS.

  i.   Kitchen layout

  ii.   Food budget

  iii. Food procurement, purchasing/ordering, and storage

  iv.   Menu and meal planning

  v.   Food preparation and service

  vi.   Kitchen and meal service staffing

  vii. Nutrition education for children, staff, and parents/guardians

  viii. Emergency preparedness for nutrition services

  ix.   Food brought from home, including food brought for celebrations

  x.   Storage, handling, and feeding of expressed human milk and ready-to-feed, concentrate, or powder formula for infants

  xi.   Age-appropriate portion sizes to meet children's nutritional needs

  xii. Age-appropriate eating utensils and tableware

  xiii. Promotion of breastfeeding and provision of community resources to support mothers who are breastfeeding

  xiv. Use and proper sanitizing of food service utensils, equipment, feeding chairs, and feeding devices

  xv.   Records of nutrition service[CFOC3 Std. 9.4.1.18]

b. **Food Purchasing and Ordering:**

_____
TITLE/NAME OF STAFF MEMBER

is responsible for ensuring that all purchased food meets the following requirements:

i. Suppliers of food and beverage must meet local, state, and federal codes. Purchased meats and poultry have been inspected and passed by federal or state inspectors.

ii. All milk products are pasteurized. Dry milk and milk products may be reconstituted in the facility for cooking purposes only, provided they are prepared, refrigerated, and stored in a sanitary manner, labeled with a date of preparation, and used or discarded within 24 hours of the date of preparation.

iii. Home-canned food; food from dented, rusted, bulging, or leaking cans; or food from cans without labels are not used.

c. **Food Service Staff and Food Safety**

i. No one with signs of illness (including vomiting, diarrhea, or open infectious skin sores) or who is known to be infected with bacteria or viruses that can be carried in food is allowed to handle food.

ii. Staff members who prepare food and change diapers or do other tasks that involve handling body fluids on the same day, complete all food preparation before doing any tasks that involve handling body fluids. Hand-washing routines followed by those who prepare food are monitored by

_____
TITLE/NAME OF STAFF MEMBER

at least once a week. In family child care homes, where there is only one adult who must handle food, assist with toileting, and perform diaper changing, as much food preparation for the day as possible is done before engaging in the routines that involve exposure to body fluids. Staff members wash their hands very carefully after assisting with toileting or diaper changing and before handling food.[CFOC3 Std. 4.9.0.2]

2. Supplies, Equipment, Furnishings, and Maintenance for Food Service

a. **Hand-washing Sinks:** Hand-washing sinks are separate from food-preparation sinks. If there is only one sink available and it is used for diapering and food preparation, the sink is disinfected before food preparation is done.

b. **Refrigerators and Freezers:** Refrigerators and freezers have thermometers that

_____
TITLE/NAME OF STAFF MEMBER

checks daily to be sure the appropriate temperature is being maintained and documents the temperature in a daily log. (See Appendix Q: Refrigerator or Freezer Temperature Log.) Refrigerators maintain temperatures at or below 41°F; freezers maintain temperatures at or below 0°F.

c. **Maintenance of Food Service Areas:**

_____
TITLE/NAME OF STAFF MEMBER

keeps food preparation, storage and service areas, and supplies and equipment clean and sanitary, according to the Food Code of the US Public Health Service, US Food and Drug Administration.[8] If local food safety standards conflict with federal recommendations, the health authority with jurisdiction determines which requirement the facility must meet.

i.   At no time are dishes, bottles, lunch boxes, or any other articles involved with food or beverages placed within a diapering or toileting area; nor are any surfaces outside the diapering or toileting area ever in contact with any object that could be contaminated by soiled diapers or soiled underclothing.

ii. Cutting boards and all other food service equipment must be made of nonporous material. Any items, including dishes and utensils, that are not washed in a dishwasher are scrubbed with hot water and detergent, then rinsed and sanitized by one of the following methods: 1) immersion in an EPA-registered chemical sanitizing solution (used according to the label on the product) and air-dried; 2) complete immersion for at least 30 seconds in hot water that is kept at 170°F, then air-dried; or 3) other methods approved by the health department. Cutting boards with crevices and cuts are not used.*CFOC3* Std. 4.9.0.10

iii. A dishwasher is used to wash dishes and food service utensils whenever possible. If dishes and utensils are washed by hand, staff members use a 3-compartment sink or 3 basins for the separate tasks of washing, rinsing, and sanitizing. A dish rack with a drain board is used for drying. No compartment used for washing dishes or utensils or food preparation is ever used for hand-washing or diaper-changing activities.*CFOC3* Stds. 4.9.0.11–4.9.0.13

d. **Food Storage, Food Temperatures, Food Preparation, and Food Service***CFOC3* Stds. 4.9.0.3–4.9.0.7

i.   This program follows the 4 basic food safety principles of the Partnership for Food Safety Education: clean, separate, cook, and chill. These principles work together to reduce the risk of food-borne illnesses.[9]

ii. Fruits and vegetables are washed thoroughly with water before use.

iii. Frozen food is defrosted in the refrigerator, under cold running water, as part of the cooking process, or by using the defrost setting of a microwave oven. Food is never defrosted by leaving it at room temperature or in standing water, a pan, or a bowl that is not inside a refrigerator.

iv. Meat, fish, poultry, milk, and egg products are placed in the coldest part of the refrigerator, not on the door, until immediately before they are used.

v.   Hot foods are kept heated over steam for no longer than 30 minutes. Then they must be covered and refrigerated or discarded. Hot foods, must be held at or above 135°F; cold foods, at or below 41°F. Cooked foods must reach the corresponding required temperatures measured with a food thermometer: ground meat, 160°F; poultry, 165°F; pork, 160°F; leftovers and casseroles, 165°F. All other foods must reach at least 145°F.

_____

TITLE/NAME OF STAFF MEMBER

checks food temperatures using a food thermometer.*CFOC3* Std. 4.9.0.3

vi. All food stored in the refrigerator except fresh, whole fruits and vegetables must be labeled with the date when the food was opened and then covered, wrapped, or placed in a container for protection from contamination. Inside a refrigerator, cooked or ready-to-eat foods are stored above raw foods that require cooking.

vii. Foods that do not require refrigerated storage are kept at least 6 inches above the floor in clean, dry, well-ventilated storerooms or other approved areas. Storage is on shelves above the floor or in another way that facilitates easy cleaning. Containers must be of a type that protects food from rodents and insects. Dry, bulk foods (eg, cereals) that are not in their original, unopened containers are stored off the floor in clean metal, glass, or food-grade plastic containers with tight-fitting covers. These containers are labeled with their contents and expiration date.

viii. Medications requiring refrigeration are stored as specified in Section 10: Health Plan.

ix. Heating of foods is done in an area that is inaccessible to children who are younger than school age. Any microwave oven must be in good condition and used only by adults and school-aged children under close supervision of an adult. Microwave heating of infant food and milk is not permitted. Food and beverages are not heated in plastic containers in a microwave oven or transferred while hot to plastic container. Plastic wrap and metal foil are not used in a microwave oven. Food heated in a microwave oven is allowed to stand for 3 to 5 minutes and stirred if it is a soft, blended food to distribute the heat in the food before it could cause burns.^{CFOC3 Std. 4.8.0.8}

x. Food that is to be served is kept covered to prevent contamination and maintained at safe food temperatures. Gloves or utensils are used instead of bare hands to touch food that is being served. Gloves are removed and discarded after they have been used to handle food.

e. Eating

i. Children who can feed themselves sit in a chair that puts the table at a level between their waist and their mid-chest and allows their feet to rest on the floor or on a firm surface so they can adjust their position while they eat.^{CFOC3 Std. 4.5.0.1}

ii. Adults who work or visit the center may not eat in the presence of children any food or beverage that does not conform to the food/feeding policies that apply to the children. Staff members are role models for children who can eat independently, conforming to the food/feeding policies that apply to the children, serving family style when possible, serving and eating the same food as the children. Nobody drinks hot beverages around the children to avoid possible burns.

iii. Children and adults always sit down to eat meals. Meals and snacks are not rushed. Children may but are not forced to remain at the table for more than a few minutes after they have finished eating.^{CFOC3 Std. 4.5.0.4}

iv. Food that has been served and not eaten from individual plates, containers, and family-style serving bowls is discarded. Cups, plates, utensils, and other food service items that fall on the floor or have been used by another person are not used without being washed. Bottles, bottle caps, and nipples are not reused without first being cleaned and sanitized.

v. Where possible, microfiber cloths that can be laundered are used instead of sponges. If a sponge is used during dish washing, it must be cleaned and disinfected between uses by being repeatedly squeezed in an EPA-registered disinfectant according to the instructions on the product label. Washable napkins and bibs are laundered after each use; tablecloths and mats are kept clean. Garbage/trash containers that hold organic material (eg, food, soiled tissues) are lined with a plastic bag and covered with a tight-fitting lid. These containers are closed after each use except when children are participating in cleanup. Garbage/trash is removed from the facility daily. Garbage/trash cans are washed and air-dried when soiled.

vi. Cleaning agents are stored separately from food. When cleaning agents or toxic materials are stored in the same room with food, these supplies are kept in a clearly labeled, locked storage cabinet that is not used for food.

D. Infant/Toddler Feeding

1. Written Feeding Instructions:

_____

TITLE/NAME OF STAFF MEMBER

obtains from the child's parent or health care professional a written description of each child's feeding history and instructions before the child enters the program. The child's teachers/caregivers review and plan to follow the instructions.

2. **Breastfeeding Is Welcome:** Staff members encourage and support breastfeeding mothers to continue breastfeeding, including feeding expressed human milk when the mother is unable to breastfeed her infant. Infant formula is not fed to a breastfed infant without the mother's written permission to do so.

   a. **Area for Breastfeeding and Pumping of Breast Milk:** This program provides a clean, private area

   ---

   LOCATION OF PRIVATE AREA

   with comfortable furniture for mothers who can come from work to breastfeed. This area has an electric outlet available to use a breast pump. Employees who are expressing milk for their babies may use this area also.

   b. **Feeding of Solid Foods:** When the infant's health care professional indicates that the baby is ready for foods in addition to human milk or infant formula, foods high in iron and zinc are gradually introduced. This introduction generally occurs between 4 and 6 months of age. Foods such as meat, beans, and eggs provide good sources of iron and zinc.

   c. **Expressed Breast Milk:** Expressed human milk must be in a sanitary BPA-free bottle or, if the milk will be fed within 72 hours of collection, in a breast milk bag/bottle system to which a nipple is or can be attached for feeding. The bottle/bag should have a water-resistant label written on with waterproof ink. The label should include the child's full name, date and time the milk was expressed, and use-by date based on the Academy of Breastfeeding Medicine Protocol #8.[10] (See Appendix R: Using Stored Human Milk.[CFOC3 Std. 4.3.1.3]) Human milk is stored immediately on arrival at the facility in a refrigerator or, if frozen, a freezer. Families are encouraged to bring human milk in volumes appropriate for a single feeding and, in addition, in some small quantities that can be used if the baby seems to want more after finishing the usual amount.

   d. **Preparing, Warming, and Feeding Human Milk:** Human milk is heated separately from other bottles in warm water or a bottle warmer, not in a slow cooker or microwave oven. Water used to heat human milk is discarded after each use. Gloves are not required for handling or feeding expressed human milk, but human milk should otherwise be treated as a body fluid. Teachers/caregivers who have openings in their skin, such as cracked skin or hangnails, should prevent contact of the human milk with their hands.

   e. **Accidental Feeding of Human Milk to the Wrong Infant:** No infant is fed the expressed human milk of another infant's mother. In the event that human milk is accidentally fed to the wrong infant, other than to a same-aged sibling, the procedure outlined in *CFOC3* will be implemented to address the potential exposure of the infant to a virus-containing fluid.[CFOC3 Std. 4.3.1.4]

3. Formula Feeding

   a. **Choice of Formula:** Infants younger than 12 months who are not fed human milk drink the formula recommended for them by their health care professionals, not cow's milk.

   b. **Receipt and Handling of Formula:** The formula must come to the facility in a factory-sealed container and be prepared according to the instructions on the formula container. An open container of ready-to-feed, concentrated formula or formula prepared from concentrated formula must be labeled with child's full name, covered, refrigerated, and discarded after 48 hours if not used. Powdered formula is stored and prepared according to the instructions on the product label.

   c. **No Solids Fed by Bottle:** No foods are mixed with formula in the bottle unless the child's health care professional provides written documentation of a medical need for this practice.

4. Feeding Procedure

   a. **When to Feed Infants:** Infants are fed on cue of hunger such as opening the mouth or making suckling sounds unless the parent and child's primary care practitioner give written instructions otherwise. These feedings are by the same teacher/caregiver whenever possible. Feedings stop when the infant seems to be satisfied or starts to fall asleep.

b. **Positioning Infants for Feedings:** Infants who are not ready to use a bottle independently while seated in a feeding chair are always held for bottle-feeding so that the infant and teacher/caregiver make eye contact during the feeding while the infant is held in the teacher's/caregiver's arms or seated on the teacher's/caregiver's lap. Bottle propping or taking bottles into sleep/rest equipment is not permitted. A child who can independently use a bottle or eat solid foods is allowed to do so only when seated or held.

c. **Use of Bottles for Infant Feedings:** Infant's bottles and foods may be warmed if the infant prefers it, but milk and food do not have to be warmed. Warming of formula and solid food is done under running warm tap water or by being put for no more than 5 minutes in a container of water that is no warmer than 120°F. Use of a microwave to warm infant formula or food is not permitted. Any formula or human milk left in a bottle from which an infant has fed is discarded by an hour after the feeding began. We _____ reuse bottles at our facility. If a bottle must be washed and reused at our facility,
DO/DO NOT
we follow our dish- and utensil-washing procedure.

d. **Progression to Use of Cups and Utensils:** Teachers/caregivers offer fluids from a cup as soon as the child seems ready to learn this drinking method, usually around 6 months of age, with a goal to wean to a cup by 12 months of age.[CFOC3 Std. 4.3.1.8] Teachers/caregivers encourage older infants and toddlers to hold and drink from a child-sized cup and to feed themselves with child-sized spoons and forks as well as to use their fingers for self-feeding. Styrofoam cups, plates, and bowls and disposable utensils are not permitted. Teachers/caregivers use small cups filled halfway to teach drinking from a cup. Teachers/caregivers discourage use of spill-resistant cups. Because prolonged contact of milk with the teeth fosters tooth decay, liquids other than water are only offered at mealtimes and snack times, with water offered as needed. No child is permitted to carry around a drinking device (ie, bottle or cup) or have such a device in any rest or exercise equipment.

e. **Solid Foods, Portions, and Appropriately Sized Tableware**
   i. Solid Foods[CFOC3 Stds. 4.3.1.11, 4.3.1.12]: Commercially prepared baby food is fed from a dish, not from the factory-sealed container. Any uneaten food in a container used for feeding is discarded. Opened containers and food prepared at home should be refrigerated and then discarded if not consumed within 24 hours. Foods are served in age-appropriate portions using plates, bowls, and cups that are sized to their servings. An individual child may have one or more additional servings of foods low in fat, sugar, and sodium as needed.

f. **Child:Staff Ratio for Feeding:** Teachers/caregivers do not feed more than one infant or supervise with more than 3 children who need close adult supervision while eating. When supervising infants and toddlers who are eating, teachers/caregivers sit within arm's reach, directly observing and communicating with the infants and toddlers who are feeding themselves.

g. **Seating for Infants and Toddler Feeding:** When high chairs or other types of infant-feeding furniture are used, the facility has on file a statement from the manufacturer that the furniture meets the ASTM standards for safety. Infant seating devices must be used with the crotch piece in place and according to the manufacturer's instructions. Teachers/caregivers use the safety straps to hold the child securely and do not rely solely on the tray for restraint. Teachers/caregivers space feeding seats so children cannot share foods. Teachers/caregivers check that a child's hands are out of the way when placing or removing the tray from the chair. Infants are not allowed to stand in the feeding chair; older children are not permitted to hang onto the feeding chair. Trays, arms, and seats of feeding chairs are cleaned and sanitized before and after each use. They are stored out of the path of doors and walkways.

h. **Meal and Snack Patterns for Toddlers:** Meals and snacks for toddlers contain the foods shown in the meal and snack patterns described in the Child and Adult Care Food Program guidelines.
   i. Food is cut up into ¼-inch pieces for infants and ½-inch pieces for toddlers to use for finger feeding by children who are 6 months and older. Round, firm, and compressible foods that might lodge in the throat of a child younger than 4 years are not permitted. These foods include but are not limited

to hot dogs, whole grapes, peanuts, popcorn, thickly spread peanut butter, hard candy, and marshmallows.[CFOC3 Std. 4.5.0.10] (See Appendix S: Fact Sheet: Choking Hazards.)

ii.   Children's hands are washed before and after feeding. Wipes or washcloths are not used instead of hand washing.

E. Preschool/School-age Feeding

1. **Foods for Meals and Snacks:** Food selections and portion sizes follow the meal and snack patterns described in the Institute of Medicine recommendations for the Child and Adult Care Food Program guidelines. Foods are planned to offer the recommended meal patterns over the course of the week, varying from day to day according to the guidelines in tables 7.1, 7.2, and 7.4 in the Institute of Medicine publication.[3]

2. **Meal Procedures**

    a.   **Hand Hygiene:** Adults and children involved with food handling, serving, or eating wash their hands before and after food-related activities.

    b.   **Child Participation in Meal Preparation:** Children help with setting the table, serving food, and cleaning the table under direct supervision of staff to ensure supervision and appropriate hand washing and adult-only sanitizing of surfaces as well as proper handling of dishes, cups, and utensils to prevent contamination.

    c.   **Grouping of Children for Meals:** Children eat in social groups with a teacher/caregiver seated with them. Children eat only when seated to decrease the possibility of choking. Teachers/caregivers eat the same food as the children, guiding and encouraging social interaction and conversation. Adults do not eat or drink anything that children are not allowed to have while the adults are in view of the children. They talk about the color, shape, size, quantity, numbers, and temperature of food as well as about events of the day.

    d.   **Family-style Meals:** Where possible, family-style service is used so children learn how to serve themselves and about table manners and socially appropriate conversation and interaction during mealtimes.

    e.   **Food Refusal:** If a child refuses to eat some type of food, the teacher/caregiver offers the same type of food again another day, up to 8 to 10 times, perhaps prepared differently or in a very small portion the next time.

    f.   **Prohibited Use of Food:** Food is not offered as a reward or denied as punishment.

F. Feeding of Children With Special Nutritional Needs

Children with special needs related to their ability to eat or a nutritional requirement must have an individual care plan that includes a written description of each child's feeding history, including prohibited foods and substitute foods where applicable, as supplied by the parent/legal guardian and the child's health care professional on admission to the program. Consultants, including nurses, nutritionists, speech therapists, occupational therapists, and physical therapists, may assist in the formation of individual feeding plans.[CFOC3 Std. 4.2.0.8] Our consultants are from

---

NAME OF CONSULTANT AND FACILITY/AGENCY WHERE THE CONSULTANT IS FROM.

G. Prevention of Obesity

This program is mindful of the relationship of feeding and other activities in the prevention of obesity. Teachers/caregivers provide opportunities for children to rest and sleep when they are tired,[CFOC3 Std. 3.1.4.4] learn about serving and choosing healthful foods and portions,[CFOC3 Stds. 2.4.1] enjoy mealtime as a socialization opportunity, avoid engaging in other activities while eating,[CFOC3 Std. 4.5.0.3] participate in recommended amounts of structured and unstructured moderate to vigorous physical activity every day,[CFOC3 Stds. 3.1.3] and limit their screen time while in child care.[CFOC3 Std. 2.2.0.3] (See Section 5: Physical Activity and Screen Time.)

H. Staff Training for Food and Feeding

Staff members who have food handling responsibilities are required to have specialized training in food service and food safety from a nutrition consultant or registered sanitarian who works in the Child and Adult Care Food Program, local health department, or local hospital or a registered dietician who works in the community.[CFOC3 Std. 1.4.5.1] Our staff members who have food handling responsibilities receive their training from

---

SOURCE OF TRAINING.

References

1. MedlinePlus. Iron deficiency anemia - children. http://www.nlm.nih.gov/medlineplus/ency/article/007134.htm. Updated February 7, 2012. Accessed August 28, 2013

2. Maguire JL, Lebovic G, Kandasamy S, et al. The relationship between cow's milk and stores of vitamin D and iron in early childhood. *Pediatrics*. 2013;131(1):e144–e151

3. Institute of Medicine of the National Academies. *Child and Adult Care Food Program: Aligning Dietary Guidance for All.* Washington, DC: Institute of Medicine of the National Academies; 2010. http://www.iom.edu/Reports/2010/Child-and-Adult-Care-Food-Program-Aligning-Dietary-Guidance-for-All.aspx. Accessed August 28, 2013

4. US Department of Agriculture Food and Nutrition Service. Child & Adult Care Food Program: meal patterns. http://www.fns.usda.gov/cnd/care/ProgramBasics/Meals/Meal_Patterns.htm. Updated January 22, 2013. Accessed August 28, 2013

5. US Environmental Protection Agency. Basic information about lead in drinking water. http://water.epa.gov/drink/contaminants/basicinformation/lead.cfm. Accessed August 28, 2013

6. Moret B. High sodium in toddler food. *The Washington Times Communities*. http://communities.washingtontimes.com/neighborhood/parenting-first-time-through/2013/mar/23/high-sodium-toddler-food. Published May 23, 2013. Accessed August 28, 2013

7. American Heart Association. Most prepackaged meals, snacks for toddlers contain too much salt [Abstract #P253]. http://newsroom.heart.org/news/most-pre-packaged-meals-snacks-for-toddlers-contain-too-much-salt. Published March 21, 2013. Accessed August 28, 2013

8. US Department of Health and Human Services. *Food Code: 2009 Recommendations of the United States Public Health Service Food and Drug Administration.* College Park, MD: US Department of Health and Human Services; 2009. http://www.fda.gov/downloads/Food/FoodSafety/RetailFoodProtection/FoodCode/FoodCode2009/UCM189448.pdf. Accessed August 28, 2013

9. Partnership for Food Safety Education. New from the Partnership for Food Safety Education. http://www.fightbac.org. Accessed August 28, 2013

10. Academy of Breastfeeding Medicine Protocol Committee. ABM clinical protocol #8: human milk storage information for home use for full-term infants (original protocol March 2004; revision #1 March 2010). *Breastfeeding Med*. 2010;5(3):127–130. Erratum. *Breastfeed Med*. 2011;6(3):159

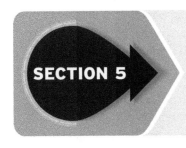

Rationale

Young children need physical activity to develop healthy bodies (brain and neurologic development, lungs, heart, muscles, bones, and appropriate weight) as well as gross motor and social skills. They sleep, learn, and exhibit greater self-regulation when physical activity is part of their daily routines. Physical activity habits developed in early childhood may last a lifetime. Young children's activity level depends on the opportunities that their teachers/caregivers and families provide for them. Because the hours spent in child care are such a large part of the child's waking hours, it is essential that child care curriculum include as much of the total time and type of physical activity children need daily as possible.

Required Action/Who Is Responsible/How Communicated

A. Encouragement of Physical Activity and Outdoor Play

1. **Role of Teachers/Caregivers:** Teachers/caregivers promote developmentally appropriate physical activity to help children (and themselves) prevent overweight/obesity and practice lifetime healthful habits.

2. **Teacher/Caregiver Participation in Physical Activity With Children:** Teachers/caregivers participate in children's active games at times when they can do so safely. Teachers/caregivers do not sit during active playtime. They prompt children to be active with comments such as "Good jump!" or "It's safe to run here." Teachers/caregivers encourage infants, toddlers, and preschool-aged children to learn basic developmentally appropriate gross motor skills by practicing physical activity and movement.

3. **Appropriate Clothing:** Appropriate clothing for all types of weather is available for each child and staff member so that outdoor play can occur except in the most extreme weather. (See sections 3.D: Required Clothing for Children and Staff Members and 5.D: Weather and Clothing for Outdoor Play.)

B. Types of and Plans for Physical Activity

1. **Types of Physical Activity**
   a. **Vigorous-Intensity Activities:** Children/adults use large muscle groups, causing rapid breathing, so it is hard for them to speak and their heart rate increases.
   b. **Moderately Intense Activities:** Children/adults use large muscle groups, causing an increased heart rate but allowing them to continue speaking.
   c. **Structured Activities:** Teachers/caregivers lead developmentally appropriate, fun, planned activities that involve all the children at their skill level in practicing motor skills.
   d. **Unstructured Activities:** Children direct their own activities; often called "free play."
   e. **Activities That Encourage Physical Activity:** Children/adults have many opportunities for exercise, such as walks in the neighborhood, dancing, going through an obstacle course, playing ball games, pulling and riding on wheeled toys, and other activities such as those suggested in reliable resources such as the *Nutrition and Physical Activity Self-Assessment*; *Color Me Healthy*; *I Am Moving, I Am Learning*; and *Motion Moments*.[1-4]

f. **Behavior and Physical Activity:** Teachers/caregivers do not use or withhold physical activity for punishment. Children whose behavior is not compatible with safe and appropriate interactions with other children have an opportunity to calm themselves before resuming cooperative play activities by staying near but not within the group of children who are playing.

2. **Frequency of Structured Activity:** Teachers/caregivers lead 2 or more structured activities or games that promote moderate to vigorous physical activity over the course of the day, indoors or outdoors. Structured activities are scheduled to come before more sedentary (nonmoving) curricular activities because children may be more attentive and learn better after periods of physical activity.

3. **Daily Active Play**_CFOC3 Std. 3.1.3.1_: All children birth to 6 years of age have continuous opportunities to develop and practice gross motor and movement skills appropriate for their age. Every day, active play includes moderate to vigorous activities such as rolling, crawling, scooting, running, climbing, dancing, hopping, galloping, skipping, and jumping. The total time for outdoor play and vigorous indoor or outdoor physical activity (adjusted for weather) is as follows:

    a. **Infants to 12 Months of Age**_CFOC3 Stds. 2.2.0.2, 3.1.3.1, 5.3.1.10_

        i. Babies who are not yet crawling spend 3 to 5 minutes (and more as the infant enjoys the activity) on their tummies interacting with their teachers/caregivers each half day while awake.

        ii. Infants are not seated for more than 15 minutes at a time, except during meals while eating or when traveling in a motor vehicle.

        iii. All infants play outdoors 2 to 3 times daily. Outdoor play for infants may include riding in a carriage or stroller in addition but not as a substitute for gross motor play outdoors. For example, infants may play on safe surfaces such as a large blanket spread on the ground outdoors with balls or other toys that encourage reaching. Examples of outdoor physical activities and play for older infants include balls to push, lie on, or kick; playing with indoor toys outside that are large enough for the baby to use to safely pull to standing position; crawling through a tube tunnel; and pushing toys across a safe surface.

    b. **Toddlers and Preschool-aged Children (12 Months to 6 Years of Age)**

        i. Children have _outdoor play_ for 60 to 90 minutes per day except in adverse weather conditions that require shorter periods outdoors. They may go outside if dressed for the weather as long as they are comfortable. (See sections 3.D: Required Clothing for Children and Staff Members and 5.D: Weather and Clothing for Outdoor Play.) If outdoor time is shortened, children have compensatory increased indoor periods of active play so the total exercise time remains the same. These activities may occur in periods that accumulate the total time for the day.

        ii. Toddlers have 60 to 90 minutes per 8-hour day of moderate to vigorous physical activity including running (prorated for children who attend the program for only part of the day—30 minutes of active play per 2 to 3 hours in the program).

        iii. Preschool-aged children have 90 to 120 minutes per 8-hour day of moderate to vigorous activities.

    c. **School-aged Children:** School-aged children have opportunities for vigorous physical activity indoors and outdoors for at least 60 minutes each day. Teachers/caregivers make plans to include all of the children in some physical activity they individually enjoy._CFOC3 Std. 2.1.4.1_

C. Equipment and Settings to Support Physical Activity

1. **Sun and Wind Protection** (See Section 8.A.11: Sun Safety): Outdoor areas provide protection from the sun with shade and protection from wind with vegetation or wind-reducing fencing.[CFOC3 Stds. 3.4.5.1, 6.1.0.7] Children use sunscreen and dress for the weather and sun exposure. (See Appendix T: Sun Safety Permission Form.)

2. **Hazards:** Outdoor and indoor areas, including surfacing and spacing under and around equipment intended for moderate to strenuous physical activity, and all equipment meet standards of the US Consumer Product Safety Commission and ASTM Standard F1487-07ae1. This facility's playgrounds had an initial inspection for safety by a playground safety inspector who is certified by the National Recreation and Park Association[5] on _____ Thereafter, outdoor playgrounds and indoor active play areas
are inspected daily by

TITLE/NAME OF STAFF MEMBER

and monthly by

TITLE/NAME OF STAFF MEMBER

to make sure there are no missing or broken parts, no protruding nuts and bolts, no rust or chipping/peeling paint, no sharp or rough edges, no splinters, and no unstable anchorages or insufficient impact-absorbing material under and around equipment on which children can climb. Outdoor play areas are free of contaminated water, animal excrement, and litter and have been tested for lead in the soil. (See Appendix O: Daily and Monthly Playground Inspection and Maintenance.) Outdoor play areas are separated a safe distance from streets, driveways, parking lots, and areas intended for other uses.[CFOC3 Stds. 6.2] Playground signs designating appropriate age and usage are posted.

3. **Equipment for Infants:** Swings, bouncy chairs, and other confining equipment are used no more than twice a day for no more than 15 minutes or not at all. Strollers may be used for walks outdoors, and feeding chairs may be used for the duration of a feeding.[CFOC3 Std. 3.1.3.1]

D. Weather and Clothing for Outdoor Play

1. **Adjustment of Outdoor Play for Weather:** Children play outdoors except when weather or air quality poses a significant health risk, defined as a wind chill factor at or below -15°F and a heat index at or above 90°F or poor air quality (eg, an ozone alert) per the National Weather Service. Scheduled outdoor play activities and times may be shortened when conditions approach these limits. Precipitation (rain or snow) does not preclude outdoor play unless a child's inner clothing becomes wet. To decide when to shorten outdoor activity, teachers/caregivers use the child care weather watch chart at www.idph.state.ia.us/hcci/common/pdf/weatherwatch.pdf.[CFOC3 Std. 3.1.3.2]

2. **Adjustment of Outdoor Play for Health Conditions:** Children who have asthma or other health conditions that are affected by weather or air quality must have a special care plan prepared in collaboration with the child's health care professional that indicates what these children can do to maximize their ability to play outdoors and when the only acceptable accommodation is an alternative to playing outdoors.

3. **Outdoor Clothing Appropriate for the Weather:** As appropriate for the weather, families must provide outdoor clothing that keeps their child dry and comfortable such as a raincoat, warm coat, boots, snow pants, mittens, and hats for cold weather or days when precipitation is expected. For sunny days, children must have lightweight clothing that is sun protective, including long-sleeved shirts and hats. (See Section 3.D. Required Clothing for Children and Staff Members and Appendix T: Sun Safety Permission Form.)

4. **Avoiding Ultraviolet Radiation Exposure:** Because ultraviolet radiation is most intense between 10:00 am and 2:00 pm, to the extent possible, outdoor play is not scheduled during these hours. If outdoor play occurs during these peak hours, children and staff members use activities in the shade, sunscreen and sun-protective clothing, and sunglasses and wide-brimmed hats that shadow the eyes, ears, face, and neck. Similar precautions are used to prevent injury from reflection of the sun by water, snow, sand, and cement at any time of day. (See Section 8.A.11: Sun Safety.)

E. Limitations for Screen Time (TV, DVD, Computers) *CFOC3* Std. 2.2.0.3

1. **Infants and Young Toddlers:** No screen time for children younger than 2 years is permitted.

2. **Children 2 Years and Older:** Children 2 years and older have no more than 30 minutes of screen time once a week while in the facility and only for educational or physical activity.

3. **Screen-free Meals and Snacks:** Children do not have any screen time during meals or snacks.

4. **Computer Time:** Computer time is no more than 15 minutes at a time except for school-aged children completing school homework assignments and for children with special health needs who require and consistently use assistive and adaptive computer technology.

5. **Content of Screen Media:** Any screen media must be free of violent, sexually explicit, stereotyped content (including cartoons), advertising, and brand placement.

References

1. Ward DS, Morris E, McWilliams C, et al. *Go NAP SACC: Nutrition and Physical Activity Self-Assessment for Child Care.* 2nd ed. Chapel Hill, NC: University of North Carolina at Chapel Hill; 2013. http://gonapsacc.org. Accessed August 5, 2013

2. North Carolina Cooperative Extension, North Carolina Division of Public Health Physical Activity & Nutrition Branch. *Color Me Healthy: Preschoolers Moving & Eating Healthy.* http://colormehealthy.com. Accessed August 5, 2013

3. US Department of Health and Human Services Administration for Children and Families Office of Head Start. *I Am Moving, I Am Learning.* http://eclkc.ohs.acf.hhs.gov/hslc/tta-system/health/Health/nutrition/nutrition%20program%20staff/iammovingiam.htm. Accessed August 5, 2013

4. National Resource Center for Health and Safety in Child Care and Early Education. *Motion Moments* [video]. http://nrckids.org/index.cfm/products/videos/motion-moments1. Accessed August 5, 2013

5. National Recreation and Park Association. http://www.nrpa.org. Accessed August 5, 2013

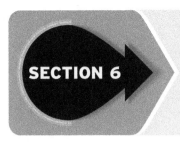

SECTION 6

Daytime Sleeping, Evening, Nighttime, and Drop-in Care

Rationale

Children need sleep for health and growth. Sleep provides the opportunity for the brain and other body tissues to repair and prepare body tissues to manage the active parts of the day. On average, children younger than 5 years sleep between 10 and 12 hours as the combined daily total of nighttime and nap time sleep. Insufficient sleep is a risk factor for overweight/obesity and behavior problems. Young children sleep and rest best at routinely scheduled times, in a relatively less stimulating place, and with consistent supervision by trusted adults. Some children are ready to nap, while others just need a quiet activity time to rest. Predictable routines help children feel comfortable. Spacing of children 3 feet apart during sleep is necessary to reduce the risk of droplet spread of infectious diseases through the air from one child to another. For infants, safe sleep practices must follow the national recommendations to reduce the risk of sleep-related deaths, including sudden infant death syndrome (SIDS) and suffocation. While swaddling of infants may help them sleep better, this practice is not recommended in child care. Swaddling can be associated with an increased risk of abnormal hip development and, if the swaddling cloth becomes loose bedding, with SIDS.^{CFOC3 Stds. 3.1.4.2, 3.1.4.4}

Required Action/Who Is Responsible/How Communicated

A. Sleep Practices

The program provides opportunities for each child to sleep and/or rest.^{CFOC3 Stds. 3.1.4.4}

1. Area/Arrangements for Sleeping and Napping

    a. **Multi-purpose Use of Rooms:** Play, eating, and sleeping may all occur in the same room (exclusive of bathrooms, kitchens, hallways, and closets), one activity after the other or at the same time, provided that the room is large enough to accommodate each activity without interfering with any other use.

    b. **Lighting and Noise in Sleeping Areas:** If possible, teachers/caregivers lower illumination and noise in the area where children are sleeping to a level that is less than what is used for active play. Lighting will be sufficient to ensure that children can be seen by the supervising teacher/caregiver and for the quiet activities that children can do while they are resting but not sleeping. (This level of lighting is about 5 foot-candles.)^{CFOC3 Stds. 5.2.2.1, 5.2.3.1}

2. Supervision of Sleeping/Resting Children

    a. **Method of Supervision:** At all times, when sleeping and resting, a teacher/caregiver who remains alert supervises children by seeing and hearing them and checking each child frequently. Another teacher/caregiver must be immediately available nearby and on the same floor, able to be summoned by the supervising teacher/caregiver in the event of an emergency.

b.   **Allowable Activities/Supervision During Rest Periods:** Children do not have to sleep, but if they do not want to sleep, they have a regular rest period when they engage in quiet play while a teacher/caregiver provides in-person supervision. Monitoring devices, if used, do not substitute for direct, in-person supervision.

TITLE/NAME OF STAFF MEMBER

ensures that all staff members, substitutes, volunteers, and families understand and accept these sleep/rest practices.

TITLE/NAME OF STAFF MEMBER

makes sure that the practices are followed in the child care facility and encourages families to continue to coordinate sleep/rest routines at home with the program's routines.

3.   **Safe Sleep Arrangements for Infants**[CFOC3 Std. 3.1.4.1]

a.   **Back-to-Sleep Positioning:** Infants younger than 12 months are placed on their backs for every sleep time unless the child's health care professional completes a signed-and-dated statement that the child requires a different sleep position.

b.   **Cribs:** Infants always sleep in a crib on a firm surface. The crib must meet current standards of the US Consumer Product Safety Commission (CPSC) and ASTM for infant sleep equipment.[CFOC3 Std. 5.4.5.2] Infants who fall asleep outside a crib are put in their cribs on their backs to continue sleeping. Only one child may sleep in the same crib at the same time. Stackable cribs are not used.

c.   **Crib Contents:** Except for a fitted sheet to cover the mattress and a pacifier, no other items are in an occupied crib with an infant, and nothing is attached to the crib or within reach of the child. Wedges, infant positioners, and blankets may not be used unless prescribed by the child's health care professional with a written note.[CFOC3 Stds. 3.1.4]

d.   **Pacifiers:** Pacifier use is allowed only during sleep time while the child is in a crib. Parents provide replacement pacifiers _____ and whenever the pacifier no longer looks the
                                        FREQUENCY
same as when it was new.

e.   **Prohibited Bedding:** Water beds and soft bedding materials such as sheepskin, quilts, comforters, pillows, crib bumpers, and granular materials (plastic foam beads or pellets) used in beanbags are not accessible to infants.

f.   **Preventing Overheating:** Infants sleep in rooms that are a comfortable temperature with clothing sufficient for warmth but that does not result in overheating. Blankets are not used. Infants are not swaddled in child care. Blanket sleepers or sleep sacks may be worn for warmth if sized to fit as garments that allow free movement of the legs and do not restrict chest movement.

g.   **Preventing Strangulation:** Nothing is tied around the child's neck or attached to the child's clothing (ie, no bibs, necklaces, garment ties, hoods, pacifier strings, or ribbons).

B. Sleep/Rest Equipment

1. **Allowable Sleep/Rest Equipment:** Sleep equipment is an individual crib, mattress pad, cot, or sleeping bag with a firm surface and of a size that accommodates the child's entire body from head to toe and separates the child from the floor. This program has written documentation from the manufacturer of the sleep equipment that it meets current standards recommended by the CPSC and ASTM and that it does not contain toxic or hazardous materials such as flame retardants that are known carcinogens now banned from children's clothing. Bunk beds are not allowed for children younger than 6 years.[CFOC3 Std. 5.4.5.5]

2. **Labeling of Sleep Equipment:** Sleep equipment is labeled with the child's full name who is the user of it until the equipment is cleaned for another child's use.

_____

TITLE/NAME OF STAFF MEMBER

check that each child's sleep equipment is labeled with the name of the one child who uses it.[CFOC3 Appendix K]

3. **Separation of Sleeping Children:** Use of space for sleeping provides 3 feet of separation between sleeping children. Walls and any floor area not concurrently occupied by furniture may be used to achieve this spacing.[CFOC3 Std. 5.4.5.1]

4. **Bedding:** The surface of the equipment in contact with the child is covered with clean, seasonally appropriate, tight-fitting covering. Bedding is not shared.

_____

FAMILIES OR TITLE/NAME OF STAFF MEMBER

wash each child's bed linen weekly or when soiled. Bed linen does not include fabrics or materials of animal origin other than wool (eg, no feathers, fur, or animal hair).

5. **Storage of Sleep Equipment and Bedding:** Sleep equipment (mattress, cot) and bedding materials (sleeping bags, sheets, pillows, blankets) are stored in such a way that there is no contact between the sleeping surfaces of one child and the sleeping surfaces of another child or with surfaces that were in contact with the floor.

C. Evening and Nighttime Care

1. **Applicable Policies:** Child care that involves dinner, evening, or nighttime care follows the same policies used for care at other times. Children who are sleeping receive the same level of supervision required for children when they are napping or resting.

2. **Evacuation Drills:** Evacuation drills occur when children are sleeping or resting, although an effort is made to choose times for the drills that are near the end of the period when children are expected to sleep.

3. **Preparation for Bed:** Stimulating activities end at least an hour before the child is expected to sleep. Calming (or appropriate) activities before bedtime include body care routines, dressing for bed, reading or telling calming stories, singing relaxing songs, and talking about the events of the day. Teachers/caregivers supervise or provide bathing or washing off before bedtime in

_____

LOCATION AND METHOD WHERE BODY HYGIENE IS DONE (EG, IN A SINK USED FOR HAND WASHING, STANDING IN A SHOWER EQUIPPED WITH A HANDHELD SHOWER HOSE).

Families provide a personal bath towel, laundered at home, and nighttime clothing for their child.

D. Drop-in Care^{CFOC3} Std. 10.4.1.1

1. **Definition of Drop-in Care:** Drop-in care is child care in which children are cared for over short periods on a one-time, intermittent, unscheduled, or occasional basis, often operated in connection with a business (eg, health club, hotel, shopping center, recreation center). This type of care may be available while parents/legal guardians are on the premises or are engaged in activities away from the child care facility. Reservations for this type of care are accepted by

    _____

    TITLE/NAME OF STAFF MEMBER

    as space and supervision are available. All policies that apply to care in this facility apply to drop-in care except those that require coordination with other programs, conferences, and maintenance of other than daily records.

2. **Intermixing of Child Groups:** To avoid an increased risk of spread of infection, intermixing children who are receiving drop-in care with those who regularly participate in child care at the facility is not allowed.

3. **Accessibility of Parents/Legal Guardians:** Parents/legal guardians must remain immediately accessible by phone or similar communication device and able to return to the facility within 30 minutes when called by a program staff member.

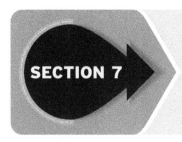

SECTION 7 **Sanitation and Hygiene**^{CFOC3} Std. 3.2

Rationale

Sanitation and hygiene are essential tools to reduce the risk of infectious diseases for children and adults, the most commonly occurring health problem in group care settings.

Required Action/Who Is Responsible/How Communicated

A. Hand Hygiene^{CFOC3} Std. 3.2.2.1

1. **Hand Hygiene Signs:** Signs are posted at each sink with times when hand hygiene is required and steps to follow.

2. **When to Practice Hand Hygiene:** All staff, volunteers, children, and visitors must perform hand hygiene at the following times:

   a. **On**

      i.   Arrival for the day

      ii. When moving from one child care group to another

      iii. When coming in from outdoors

   b. **Before and After**

      i.   Preparing, eating, and handling food or beverages or feeding a child

      ii. Giving medication or applying a medical ointment or cream in which a break in the skin (eg, sores, cuts, scrapes) may be encountered

      iii. Playing, wading, or swimming in water that is used by more than one person

   c. **After**

      i.   Diapering, using the toilet, or helping a child use the toilet

      ii. Handling body fluids (eg, urine, feces, mucus, blood, vomit); wiping noses, mouths, and sores; handling mouthed toys; checking the need for a diaper change by touching the inside of the diaper or touching any clothing contaminated by stool, urine, or body fluids

      iii. Cleaning or handling garbage

      iv. Handling animals or cleaning up animal waste or habitats

      v.   Playing in sand or other sensory table materials, on wooden play structures, or outdoors

3. Hand Washing

    a. Preference for Hand Washing: Hand washing is the preferred way for all staff members, volunteers, children, and visitors to perform hand hygiene.

    b. Method for Hand Washing at a Sink:

        i.   Turn on water to a comfortable temperature (60°F–110°F).

        ii.   Moisten hands with water and apply liquid (not antibacterial) soap.

        iii.   With hands out of the water, lather all skin surfaces and nails with soap and water. Try to achieve the recommended lathering time of 20 seconds. (Sing or say twice "Happy Birthday to You"; "Twinkle, Twinkle, Little Star"; or a jingle of comparable length such as, "Wash, wash, wash your hands; play this handy game; scrub and rub; rub and scrub; germs go down the drain" sung twice to the tune of "Row, Row, Row Your Boat"). Include between fingers, under and around nail beds, backs of hands, and any jewelry. *Note:* Nails must be kept short; acrylic nail covers and wearing of chipped nail polish is not permitted. Because participation in child care activities is likely to chip nail polish, wearing of nail polish is discouraged.

        iv.   Rinse hands well under running water with fingers down so water flows from wrist to fingertips.

        v.   Leave the water running while drying hands with a disposable paper towel, a single-use or individually labeled single-person cloth towel, or a drying device approved by local health authorities. Drying devices are used only in situations in which faucet taps turn off automatically so that the user doesn't touch the faucet once hands have been washed.

        vi.   Use a towel to turn off the faucet and, if inside a toilet room with a closed door, to open the door. Discard the towel in a lined trash container, place a single-use towel in a laundry hamper, or hang an individually labeled cloth towel to dry.

        vii.   Apply hand lotion, if needed, to prevent dry, cracked skin.

    c. Alternate Hand Wash for Children Unable to Stand or Be Held at a Sink: If a child cannot stand at a sink and is too heavy to hold for hand washing at the sink, the teacher/caregiver may use this method. It is less satisfactory than hand washing at a sink.

        i.   Use disposable wipes or a damp paper towel moistened with a drop of liquid soap to clean the child's hands.

        ii.   Wipe the child's hands with a paper towel wet with clear water.

        iii.   Dry the child's hands with a fresh paper towel.

4. Hand Sanitizers[CFOC3 Std. 3.2.2.5]: The use of alcohol-based hand sanitizers is an acceptable alternative to traditional hand washing with soap and water by children older than 24 months and by adults on hands that are not visibly soiled.

a. Acceptable Conditions for Use of Hand Sanitizers:

        i.   Alcohol-based hand sanitizers are those with 60% to 95% alcohol.

        ii.   Any visible soil must be removed by hand washing or a wet wipe before applying the sanitizer.

        iii.   To avoid ingestion, contact with eyes and mucous membranes, and inhalation of fumes, alcohol-based hand sanitizer dispensers are not accessible to children younger than 6 years.

        iv.   Use of hand sanitizers requires 1:1 supervision by an adult to dispense and making sure that the chemical is used according to the directions on the product label. School-aged children may use hand sanitizers with close teacher/caregiver supervision.

        v.   Users should pay special attention to the time the skin must stay wet with the hand sanitizer before being allowed to air-dry.

b. **Procedure for Using a Hand Sanitizer:**

i. Dispense the amount recommended by the manufacturer of the alcohol-based sanitizer.

ii. Rub hands together, distributing sanitizer to all hand and finger surfaces and keeping hand surfaces wet for the time specified on the product label.

iii. Allow hands to air-dry.

B. Diapers, Clothing, and Changing Areas Soiled by Body Fluids*CFOC3* Std. 3.2.1

1. **Type of Diapers:** This facility allows use of disposable absorbent diapers that prevent spills of feces or urine. Exceptions require documentation by the child's health care professional of the medical reason for using cloth diapers. If cloth diapers are used, they must meet the following criteria: the diaper has an absorbent inner lining completely contained within an outer covering made of waterproof material that prevents the escape of feces and urine, or the cloth diaper is adherent to a waterproof cover.

2. **Soiled Diapers, Training Pants, and Other Clothing Soiled by Body Fluids:** No soiled clothing has its contents dumped or is rinsed at the child care facility. Disposable diapers are placed in a hands-free, plastic-lined, lidded container. Soiled cloth items are completely contained in a non-permeable, sealed plastic bag before being moved from the location where the child is being changed. Soiled cloth diapers may be stored in a labeled container with a tight-fitting lid provided by an accredited commercial diaper service. Otherwise they are placed in a sealed plastic bag for removal from the facility by an individual child's family. All soiled cloth items are stored in

---

LOCATION INACCESSIBLE TO CHILDREN

until delivered to the parent/guardian at the end of the child care day.

3. **Changing Location:** Diapering and changing of soiled clothing are done only in an area designated for these activities. The changing procedure is posted in the changing area and followed for all changes done in this facility by staff or family members. The signage is simple, mostly illustrations rather than many words, and in the languages of those who do changing in the facility. Surfaces in the designated areas are kept clean, waterproof, and free of cracks, tears, and crevices. (For more information about the most recently updated diapering poster, visit www.ecels-healthychildcarepa.org/news/item/464-diapering-poster-procedure-revised-may-2013.)

4. **Separation of Food Preparation From Items Soiled by Body Fluids:** Food handling is not permitted in areas designated for changing. If possible, staff members who change diapers or soiled clothing are not involved in food preparation for the rest of the day after they have been involved in changing diapers or clothing soiled with feces or urine.

5. **Disinfecting Changing Surfaces:** Anyone who changes children's diapers or clothing soiled by urine or feces will disinfect the contaminated surfaces with a US Environmental Protection Agency (EPA)-registered disinfectant suitable for the surface material that is being disinfected to maintain surfaces in a sanitary condition. Dilution of cleaning and disinfecting solutions is done in

---

LOCATION OF A WELL-VENTILATED AREA, AWAY FROM THE CLASSROOM.

Diluted solutions are kept in the changing area so they are accessible to the teacher/caregiver but out of reach of any child.

6. **Checking Children for Need to Be Changed:** Hourly, children who have not yet mastered reliable use of the toilet are checked for the need to be changed by external appearance and smell. At least every 2 hours, children who wear diapers or training pants have their diapers or training pants removed to check for a need to be changed or use the toilet.[CFOC3 Std. 3.2.1.3]

7. **Procedure for Changing/Checking Diapers or Clothing Soiled by Body Fluids**[CFOC3 Std. 3.2.1.4]

   a. **Monitoring for Use of Correct Changing Procedure:**

   _____

   TITLE/NAME OF STAFF MEMBER

   evaluates compliance with the following changing procedures specified in c.iii at least

   _____

   FREQUENCY OF EVALUATION.

   b. **Supervision of Children During Changing:** Children being changed are supervised by touch at all times when they are on an elevated surface. Safety straps or harnesses are not present in the changing area because they become contaminated during a change. If an emergency arises, teachers/caregivers bring the child from any elevated surface to the floor or take the child with them.

   c. **Changing Procedure**

      i. **Get Organized**
         - Before bringing the child to the changing area, perform hand hygiene if hands were soiled by checking inside a child's diaper.
         - Cover the changing surface with nonabsorbent paper. (If the child is changed lying down, the paper should extend from the child's shoulders to beyond the child's feet. If the child is changed standing up, use enough paper to extend an arm's reach around the child.)
         - Remove the following items from containers and place them away from the child's reach, on a part of the changing area that is likely to stay clean during the change:
           – Unused diaper, clean clothes
           – Wipes
           – A plastic bag for any soiled clothes or cloth diapers
           – Dab of diapering cream on facial or toilet tissue
           – Disposable gloves, if to be used
         - Make sure the disinfecting solution to be used after the change is available to the adult doing the change but inaccessible to any child.

      ii. **Prepare the Child for the Change**
         - Bring the child to the changing surface, keeping soiled clothing away from the adult and off any surfaces that cannot be easily cleaned and disinfected after the change. Keep a hand on the child at all times.
         - Undress the child. If the child's feet cannot be kept from touching soiled clothing or skin, remove the child's shoes and socks. Remove bottom outer clothing and any other soiled clothing. If the child is able, have the child hold unsoiled upper-body clothing up away from the soiled area of the body.
         - Put any soiled clothing in the plastic bag.

iii. **Remove Soiled Diaper/Underclothing and Clean Child's Skin**

- Unfasten and check the diaper/underclothing. If the child was wearing a disposable diaper or training garment that has pull-apart sides, leave it where soiled wipes can be put in it or put the soiled diaper or training garment and each wipe immediately into the plastic-lined, hands-free covered can. Close any safety pins immediately and keep them out of the child's reach. (Teachers/caregivers should never hold pins in their mouth.)
- Clean the child's skin that was in contact with urine or feces.
- Lift child's legs and clean bottom from front to back. Use fresh wipe each time.
- Keep a hand on the child. Put the soiled wipes into the soiled diaper/training pants and fold the soiled surface of the diaper/training pants inward. Then put these into a plastic-lined, hands-free, lidded container. Alternately, dispose of each of these items individually when done with them. Cloth diapers go into the can provided by the commercial diaper service. Articles that get laundered at home go into a tightly sealed plastic bag, avoiding squeezing or touching soiled surfaces, and then can be put in a separate lidded, plastic-lined, hands-free covered container.
- If the disposable paper is soiled, use a corner of the paper to fold the clean side of the paper back under the child's bottom. The adult removes the disposable gloves by pinching the soiled surface of the first glove with the other hand, holding the soiled glove in the palm of the still-gloved hand. Then the adult puts a bare finger into the inside of the cuff of the second glove, pulling it off and over the glove in the palm of the glove so soiled surfaces are contained inside the second glove. Dispose of the gloves as done for the wipes. Use a separate clean wipe to clean the child's hands (that may have strayed into soiled areas) and another fresh wipe to clean the adult's hands. *(This is the end of the soiled part of the procedure).*

iv. **Prepare to Put on Clean Clothing:** All contaminated materials should be in the hands-free, lidded, plastic-lined covered container or bagged in plastic to be sent out of the facility for laundering. Hands have been wiped; the soiled area of the disposable paper is folded on itself, so a clean surface is ready for the clean steps that follow.

v. **Dress the Child:** Put on a clean diaper or underclothes and dress the child.

- Slide a fresh diaper under the child or fresh underclothing on the child's ankles.
- Use a facial or toilet tissue or wear a clean, disposable glove to apply any necessary diaper cream for which the facility has a signed note giving parental request and permission to use it. Discard the tissue or glove in a plastic-lined, hands-free covered can.
- Fasten the diaper or pull up the fresh underclothing and finish dressing the child. Older children may help put their clean clothes on with coaching from the teacher/caregiver. For this clean part of the change, do not stand the child on the diapering surface to avoid contaminating the bottom of the child's shoes, which then spread contamination around the room.

vi. **Wash the Child's Hands Before Returning the Child to a Supervised Area**

- Use soap and warm water, between 60°F and 120°F, at a sink to wash the child's hands.
- Use a disposable wipe to clean the child's hands only if the child cannot be held or is unable to stand at the sink.
- Help the child leave the changing area and go to supervised play.

vii.   **Clean and Disinfect Changing Surfaces**
- Put the disposable changing paper in a plastic-lined, hands-free covered can.
- If clothing was soiled, securely tie the plastic bag used to store and send it home.
- If changing surfaces are visibly soiled, use paper towels to wash surfaces with detergent and water, then rinse with water.
- Wet the entire changing surface with a disinfectant as a closely directed spray or poured solution. Use an EPA-registered disinfectant according to the product label. Note the required contact time and whether the EPA-registered product requires rinsing with water after the required contact time.

viii.   **Finish Up**
- Perform hand hygiene by washing hands at a sink or using alcohol-based hand sanitizer.
- Record in a log accessible to the family the time of the diaper change, what was in the diaper or soiled clothing, and any problems, such as a loose stool, an unusual odor, blood in the stool, or any skin irritation.
- Dry off the changing surface if it doesn't dry by itself before the next change.

C. Toileting

1. Location of Toilets: Toilets for adults who care for infants are located

_____
LOCATION IN/NEAR INFANT ROOMS

to minimize their absence from supervising the children. Toilets for toddlers are located

_____
LOCATION AS CLOSE AS POSSIBLE, PREFERABLY ADJACENT TO THE ROOMS WHERE THE CHILDREN ARE IN CARE.

Toilets for preschool- and school-aged children[CFOC3 Std. 5.4.1.2] are located

_____
LOCATION AS CLOSE AS POSSIBLE, NEAR THE ENTRANCE TO THEIR ROOMS AND NEAR THE ENTRANCE TO THE BUILDING FROM THE PLAYGROUND.

Toilet areas are not used for any activity other than toileting. No cooking, food preparation, eating, or any activity other than toileting and hand washing is permitted in toileting areas. Privacy and separate toilets for girls and boys are available for children who are 6 years or older at

_____
LOCATION AS CLOSE AS POSSIBLE, NEAR THE ENTRANCE TO THEIR ROOMS.

2. Adaptation of Toilets for Independent Use: Children use

_____
INDICATE WHETHER THE ADAPTATION IS A CHILD-SIZED TOILET, A NONSLIP PLASTIC STEP, OR A TOILET SEAT ADAPTER

with a nonporous surface that is easy to wash and disinfect.

_____
TITLE/NAME OF STAFF MEMBER

ensures that toilet paper and holders are available where children can easily reach them while seated at the toilet and that paper towels and soap dispensers are easily reached while standing at the sink. Disposable, nonporous gloves are within easy reach of teachers/caregivers in the toilet area.

3. **Potties (Potty Chairs, Training Chairs, Non-flushing Toilets):** These are not permitted because of the risk of spreading infectious diseases. If an exception is made, the potty is individually assigned, used, and stored only in the toilet room. After each use,

_____

TITLE/NAME OF STAFF MEMBER

empties the potty into the toilet and cleans and disinfects it in a utility sink designated only to be used for cleaning and sanitizing potties in _____The utility sink must be cleaned and

LOCATION.

disinfected after each use.[CFOC3 Std. 5.4.1.7]

4. **Monitoring of Toileting Procedures:**

_____

TITLE/NAME OF STAFF MEMBER

monitors toileting areas at least weekly to ensure that proper hand washing and cleaning procedures are followed.

5. **Privacy for Toileting:** Younger children who can demonstrate an ability to use the toilet properly and independently and who request privacy are allowed to use the toilet without adult assistance but with supervision immediately outside the toilet cubicle/room. Teachers/caregivers open a private toilet from the outside if the child needs help.[CFOC3 Std. 5.4.1.3] Infants and toddlers are always under sight-and-sound supervision and not allowed unattended access to toilet areas.[CFOC3 Std. 5.4.1.4] Children younger than 6 years and older children who require assistance are accompanied to the toilet by an adult.

6. **Maintenance of Toilet Areas:**

_____

TITLE/NAME OF STAFF MEMBER

checks toilets after each use to be sure the toilets are kept visibly clean. Toilets should not be shared by different groups of toddlers and preschool-aged children. Daily, and when toilet area surfaces are visibly soiled,

_____

TITLE/NAME OF STAFF MEMBER

cleans and disinfects toilets and all other surfaces in the toilet area. Staff members who clean toilets wear nonporous gloves when doing this cleaning, followed by hand washing. They do not prepare food for the rest of the program day after cleaning toilets.[CFOC3 Std. 5.4.1.8] (See Section 7.C.3 for maintenance of potty chairs/non-flushing toilets.)

D. Oral Hygiene

See Section 10.B: Oral Health.

E. Facility Cleaning, Sanitizing, and Disinfecting

Cleaning means removing visible soil. *Sanitizing* means reducing the number of germs that can cause disease to a level generally accepted as safe by public health authorities. *Disinfecting* means nearly, but not completely, eliminating germs that can cause disease.

1. **Routine Schedule:** This facility follows the schedule for routine cleaning, sanitizing, and disinfecting of surfaces and objects outlined in Appendix U: Routine Schedule for Cleaning, Sanitizing, and Disinfecting, [CFOC3 Stds. 3.3] using products as outlined in Section 8.A.2: Cleaning/Sanitizing/Disinfecting and Other Maintenance; Toxic Supplies and Pesticides.

2. **General Cleaning Personnel:** The people who clean this facility are

   _____

   INDICATE WHO DOES THE CLEANING BY TITLE/NAME OF STAFF MEMBER OR NAME OF JANITORIAL SERVICE.

   As a life-skills learning activity, children may help with cleaning routines for areas they use that are not expected to involve children touching body fluids of others. They may use water and paper towels to clean but no cleaning products. Children must not be nearby, and the area must be well ventilated if anyone is using volatile or potentially hazardous cleaning products.

   _____

   TITLE/NAME OF STAFF MEMBER

   is responsible for supervision to be sure that required routines are done in this facility.

3. **Personnel Responsible for Cleaning and Sanitizing Toys:**

   _____

   TITLE/NAME OF STAFF MEMBER

   cleans and sanitizes toys. No toys that might be mouthed or objects intended to be placed in the mouth are allowed if they cannot be cleaned and sanitized by being washed in a mechanical dishwasher, using the hand-washing procedure for food service utensils, or by being laundered.[CFOC3 Std. 3.3.0.2]

4. **Bedding:** Each child's bedding is stored individually in

   _____

   SPECIFY A BAG, CUBBY, OR OTHER CONTAINER

   separate from bedding of other children.

   _____

   FACILITY OR FAMILY

   launder bedding that touches a child's skin weekly and before being used by another child.[CFOC3 Std. 3.3.0.4]

5. **Water Play:** Water play equipment (eg, water table, wading pool) and toys used for water play are closely supervised when being used. Such equipment is supplied with free-flowing, fresh, drinkable water that drains out as fresh water comes in or is filled with fresh, drinkable water immediately before designated children begin a play activity with the equipment. The water is changed before children other than those for whom the equipment was first filled with fresh water come to play.[CFOC3 Std. 6.2.4.2]

6. **Spills:** When a spill occurs, the area is made inaccessible to children and

_____

TITLE/NAME OF STAFF MEMBER

is notified about the need for cleanup. When surfaces are soiled by body fluids or other potentially infectious material, they are cleaned with detergent and water, rinsed with water to remove all organic material, and disinfected using a (nontoxic) EPA-registered disinfectant, strictly following the label directions. Alternatively they may be disinfected with a diluted solution of non–EPA-registered household bleach according to the instructions on the Centers for Disease Control and Prevention (CDC) Web site, www.cdc.gov.

7. **Rugs/Carpets:** Rugs that cannot be laundered in a clothes-washing machine are not used. Washable rugs are machine washed whenever they are soiled and monthly.

8. **Instruction of Staff for Cleaning, Sanitizing, and Disinfecting:**

_____

TITLE/NAME OF STAFF MEMBER

arranges for at least annual instruction for all staff members who are responsible for cleaning/sanitizing/disinfecting and those who may use these procedures occasionally. The instruction includes information required by the US Occupational Safety and Health Administration (OSHA) about the use of any chemical agents with a review and explanation of the Safety Data Sheets for these chemicals.

F. Exposure to Blood and Other Potentially Infections Materials

1. Risk Reduction

a. **Exposure to Cuts or Sores:** Open cuts or sores on children or staff members are kept covered. If it is not possible to cover open cuts or sores, exclusion may be required until healing occurs.

b. **Response to Exposure to Body Fluids:** Whenever a child or staff member comes into contact with any body fluids, the exposed area is washed immediately with soap and warm water, rinsed, and dried with paper towels. When a staff person or child comes into contact with blood (eg, staff member provides first aid for a child who is bleeding) or is exposed to blood (eg, blood from one person enters the cut or mucous membrane of another person), the staff person should inform

_____

TITLE/NAME OF STAFF MEMBER

immediately. If blood splashes into the mouth, nose, or eyes, these surfaces should be rinsed for at least 15 minutes with water. The procedure thereafter follows guidance obtained by contacting

_____

NAME/TITLE/SECTION/PHONE NUMBER OR E-MAIL ADDRESS AT HEALTH DEPARTMENT TO CONTACT.

2. **Standard Precautions to Avoid Exposure to Body Fluids:** Staff members follow Standard Precautions developed by the CDC, adapted for child care. These are consistent with Universal Precautions required by OSHA related to prevention of blood-borne infections. Adaptation of Standard Precautions for child care requires use of gloves only if blood or blood-containing or infectious body fluids might contact hands or splash into the mouth, eyes, or nose.*CFOC3 Std. 3.2.3.4, CFOC3 Appendix L*. Gowns and masks are not required unless blood might spray into the mouth, nose, or eyes. Surfaces that might come in contact with infectious body fluids must be disposable or able to be disinfected.

   a. **Spills of Body Fluids:** Spills of vomit, urine and feces, blood, and injury and tissue discharges are cleaned and disinfected as for the procedure for diaper-changing tables.

   b. **Disposal of Contaminated Materials:** Contaminated materials are disposed of in a plastic bag with a secure tie or closure (ie, gloves, paper towels, or other materials used to wipe up body fluids).

   c. **Contaminated Articles That Can Be Used Again:** Reusable rugs and other fabric articles are laundered. Brushes, brooms, dustpans, and mops used to clean up body fluids are washed with detergent, rinsed, and soaked in a disinfecting solution according to instructions on the product label. Items such as mop heads and reusable rags are washed with hot water and detergent in the washing machine. All items are hung off the floor or ground to dry. Equipment used for cleaning is stored safely out of children's reach in an area ventilated to the outside.

3. **Soiled Clothing:** Clothing items soiled with body fluids are put into a closed plastic bag and sent home with the child's parent/legal guardian or, if adult clothing, sent home for the staff member to launder. A full change of clothing, including shoes, is kept in the facility for children in care as well as for staff members.

4. **Hand Hygiene After Handling Contaminated Materials:** Hands are always washed after handling soiled laundry or equipment and after removing gloves.

5. **Blood-borne Pathogen Exposure Plan:**

   _____

   TITLE/NAME OF STAFF MEMBER

   is responsible for developing the blood-borne pathogens (BBP) exposure plan required by OSHA, ensuring all staff members learn how to protect themselves from exposure to body fluids and follow requirements for immunization against hepatitis B of staff members whose jobs include the risk of exposure to blood (eg, by providing first aid). The BBP exposure plan confirms the requirements reflected in the OSHA model plan found at www.osha.gov/Publications/osha3186.pdf.

G. Animals, Including Pets

1. **Allowable Animals:** The only allowable animals that may have contact with children and adults in our program indoors or outdoors are those that are older than 1 year; are not aggressive; are adapted to be with young children; show no evidence of disease, fleas, ticks, or poor health; are fully immunized; and are on an intestinal parasite control program. Acceptable pets are one of the following types: dogs (except for wolf-dog hybrids), cats, ungulates (eg, cows, sheep, goats, pigs, horses), rabbits, and rodents as indicated by a time-specified current certificate from the animal's veterinarian. Fish are allowed if they are inaccessible to children.*CFOC3 Stds. 3.4.2.1, 3.4.2.2*

2. **Supervision of Animal Contact:** Teachers/caregivers supervise all contact between animals and children closely enough to ensure humane and safe treatment of the animal, prevent close contact between the animal and children's faces, and immediately remove the child if the animal seems distressed. When an animal is not in its cage, it must be controlled by a responsible adult. Toys used by animals are kept separate from children's toys. Children are not allowed to feed animals directly from their hands or have access to animal food, food

dishes, animals that are feeding, or litter boxes or habitats that contain feces or urine. No food or beverages or any dishware or utensils involved in feeding people are allowed in animal areas, and no animal is allowed in food preparation areas, storage and eating areas, hand-washing areas, supply rooms, or areas where children routinely play or gather such as sandboxes and playgrounds.

3. **Cleaning Animal Habitats:** Pet dishes may not be washed or filled in any sink used for human food preparation. Animal living areas must be enclosed and their waste cleaned out by an adult who is not a food handler or who has completed food-handling duties for the day. Animal waste is removed immediately from children's areas and disposed of in a sealed plastic bag or container or put into a flushing toilet. Pregnant women will not be allowed to handle cat waste or litter. Only adults may clean aquariums. Aquarium cleaning is done without dumping water into any sink used for food preparation or drawing drinking water. Hand washing immediately follows anyone's contact with an animal or its habitat.[CFOC3 Std. 3.4.2.3]

4. **Supervision of Animal Care in the Facility:**

_____

TITLE/NAME OF STAFF MEMBER

is responsible for checking that the appropriate care instructions for pets are followed.

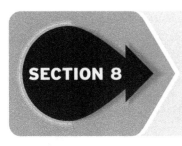

SECTION 8 Environmental Health

Rationale

"…[C]hildren generally spend most of their active, awake time at schools and child care facilities. Children are especially sensitive to contamination, for several reasons. First, children are biologically more vulnerable than adults since their bodies are still growing and developing. Second, children's intake of air and food is proportionally greater than that of adults. For example, relative to body weight, a child may breathe up to twice as much air as adults do; this increases their sensitivity to indoor air pollutants. In particular for younger children, the inhalation and ingestion of contaminated dust is a major route of exposure due to their frequent and extensive contact with floors, carpets, and other surfaces where dust gathers, such as windowsills, as well as their high rate of hand-to-mouth activity. Lastly, children have many years of future life in which to develop disease associated with exposure."[1]

Toxicity is related to amount and type of a potentially harmful exposure. A wise approach to environmental health risks is to use peer-reviewed, scientific evidence, employing reasonable precautions in situations in which evidence suggests that the magnitude of risk justifies the difficulty of taking preventive action.

Required Action/Who Is Responsible/How Communicated

A. Avoiding Significant Noxious/Toxic/Infectious Disease Environmental Exposures

1. Air Quality/Temperature/Humidity

a. **Heating and Cooling Equipment:** Maintenance of heating and cooling equipment includes an inspection and repairs[CFOC3 Std. 5.2.1.3] recommended by

---

NAME AND CONTACT INFORMATION FOR THE HVAC CONTRACTOR RECOMMENDED BY THE LOCAL CHAPTER OF THE AMERICAN SOCIETY OF HEATING, REFRIGERATING AND AIR-CONDITONING ENGINEERS (ASHRAE). (SEE WWW.ASHRAE.ORG.)

---

b. **Ventilation:** All rooms are ventilated with fresh outdoor air as much as possible with the rate and method determined by our HVAC contractor according to national standards for the occupancy of the room. For child care, fresh air ventilation should be between 15 and 60 cu ft per minute per person. American National Standards Institute (ANSI)/ASHRAE 62.1-2007 calls for 10 cu ft per minute per person plus 0.18 cu ft per minute per square foot of space.[CFOC3 Std. 5.2.1.1] To minimize drawing in pollutants from outdoors, the air intakes for building ventilation are located

---

LOCATION.

---

c. **Humidity and Temperature:** Draft-free mechanical systems are used to maintain indoor humidity in the range of 30% to 50% to prevent mold growth and avoid excessive loss of body moisture. Temperatures are kept at 68°F to 75°F in cooler months and 74°F to 82°F in warmer months as measured by durable digital thermometers in each room at child height.^{CFOC3 Stds. 5.2.1.2, 5.2.1.9}

d. **Odor Control:** Ventilation, cleaning, and use of closed containers control odors. No air fresheners, scented products, or deodorizers other than baking soda are used.^{CFOC3 Std. 5.2.1.6}

e. **Outdoor Air Quality:**

_____
TITLE/NAME OF STAFF MEMBER

checks the Air Quality Index (AQI) daily on the US Environmental Protection Agency (EPA) Web site at www.epa.gov/airnow, by using media reports, or by receiving alerts available by signing up at www.enviroflash.info. If the AQI is between 0 and 50, all children may play outside. If it is higher than 50, teachers/caregivers check special care plans for children with such plans to see which children need an alternate activity indoors for the current AQI level.^{CFOC3 Std. 3.1.3.3}

f. **Tobacco Smoke Prohibited:** Smoking is not allowed anywhere on the premises or in vehicles used to transport children at any time. To prevent thirdhand smoke exposure, anyone who smokes is required to keep and wear clean clothing at the facility that has not been worn when the individual was smoking and was not kept in an environment where smoking occurs.^{CFOC3 Stds. 3.4.1.1, 9.2.3.15}

2. Cleaning/Sanitizing/Disinfecting and Other Maintenance; Toxic Supplies and Pesticides

a. **Integrated Pest Management**

i.   All pest control activities use the techniques described as integrated pest management and detailed by the EPA at www.epa.gov/pesticides/ipm/index.htm. The least toxic, most effective approaches to cleaning/disinfecting/sanitizing and controlling pests are used in this facility. When chemicals are needed, if possible, this program uses products labeled with the EPA Design for the Environment or the logo of a third-party certifier (ie, Green Seal or EcoLogo).

ii. Integrated pest management for this program includes keeping pests out of the facility by removing food (ie, keep kitchen area clean and food items in sealed containers), water (ie, fix leaky pipes), and shelter (ie, organize clutter, seal gaps) for pests. Mechanical exclusion of pests is the first approach. Pesticides are used only as a last resort when pests are present and cannot be controlled by mechanical means and less harmful pesticides (ie, gels or baits rather than broadcast sprays).

iii. If, as a last resort, pesticide applications are needed, at least 3 days prior to the pesticide application,

_____
TITLE/NAME OF STAFF MEMBER

notifies all staff members, families, and visitors to the facility about the plan. Notification involves sending a letter, an e-mail, or other individual communication that includes the name of the pesticide, Safety Data Sheet (SDS) for that product, and where and when it will be applied. In addition, this information will be posted in an easily viewed location in the facility and remain posted for 2 days after the treatment.^{CFOC3 Std. 5.2.8.1}

iv. If, as a last resort, pesticide sprays are used, food and mouthed items are removed before spraying; tabletops and surfaces where children eat and play or food is prepared are removed or covered. Children are not allowed to reenter an area where a pesticide was applied for at least 7 hours or as long as stated on the pesticide product label.

v.   Any contractor and anyone who applies pesticide or who provides any type of pest-control services for this facility must be licensed by the state and certified as a pest control operator and have successfully completed training from state-recognized sources about how to use integrated pest management approaches.

_____

TITLE/NAME OF STAFF MEMBER

directly observes the contractor's work in this facility to ensure that the contractor's staff performs in accordance with the pest control policies of this facility.

vi.   All staff members in this facility are required to receive integrated pest management training. (See *Integrated Pest Management: A Toolkit for Early Care and Education Programs* at www.ucsfchildcarehealth.org/html/pandr/trainingcurrmain.htm.)

b.   Products Used in the Facility for Maintenance

i.   As few different maintenance products as possible are used in this facility.

ii.   All staff members and contractors who use any cleaning/sanitizing/disinfecting or maintenance chemicals/supplies or pesticides read and follow the label instructions on EPA-registered products.

_____

TITLE/NAME OF STAFF MEMBER

directly observes the use of potentially toxic chemicals by program staff and contractors to ensure that they are used as required on the product label and in these policies. Toxic products that leave a residue are not applied to surfaces that children are likely to touch, or any residue is removed. No toxic product may be applied when children are present in the area.

iii.   All fruits and vegetables are thoroughly cleaned using free-flowing water and where practical, a vegetable brush as the first step in food preparation.

iv.   Safety Data Sheets are available for all products used in this facility

_____

WHERE SDSs ARE FOUND IN THE FACILITY.

v.   Staff members and contractors must follow written procedures for cleaning and maintenance found in

_____

WHERE PROCEDURES ARE KEPT AND ACCESSIBLE TO STAFF.

vi.   Only products that have low volatile organic compounds (VOCs) (ie, products that do not emit significant amounts of chemical into the air) are used in this facility.

vii.   No aerosols of any kind are used in this facility.

viii.   All potentially toxic chemicals are inaccessible to children, stored in a manner that they are not likely to tip over, and applied only when children are not near enough to have contact with or inhale the product.

ix.   All flammable products, including bulk supplies of hand sanitizer, are stored where they are inaccessible to children, in

_____

LOCATION OF A SEPARATE BUILDING.

In this location, they are protected from excess heat or sources of ignition and kept locked except to access these materials.[CFOC3 Std. 5.5.0.5]

3. **Water Quality** (See also Section 2.D: Swimming, Wading, Gross Motor Water Play.)

   a. **Water Supply:** Our facility uses

   _____

   SPECIFY THE PUBLIC/PRIVATE SOURCE

   for our water supply. Our water meets EPA standards for drinking water from an approved source as confirmed by the local health department on

   _____ The water _____ contain appropriate amounts of fluoride to
   DATE.   DOES/DOES NOT

   prevent tooth decay. In addition, our water was tested for the presence of lead and copper that might come from our pipes _____ For well water: Our well water is tested annually.
   DATE WHEN TESTED.

   The results[CFOC3 Stds. 5.2.6.1–5.2.6.3] are on file

   _____

   WHERE THE RESULTS ARE FILED.

   b. **Communal Water Play:** If children engage in communal water play in water tables or unfiltered wading pools where more than one child plays in the same water, the container and toys used in the activity are disinfected before each use of the table or pool and staff members supervise the water play closely to be sure no child drinks the water or has any contact between body fluids (from the child's nose, mouth, or eye) and the water. An alternative to these precautions is to give each child a personal basin of water for play or allow the children to play in a sprinkler. Before children play in a communal water table, be sure they wash their hands, then supervise the activity closely. The program _____ include use
   DOES/DOES NOT

   of swimming or wading pools. If used, these pools meet the standards of the health department and the water is tested _____ to be sure it is safe with a ph between 7.2 and 7.8 and chlorine or
   FREQUENCY OF TESTING

   bromine present in a safe level of 1 to 3 ppm for chlorine and 1 to 6 ppm for bromine.[CFOC3 Std. 6.3.4.1]

4. **Noise:** Noise levels in occupied areas must be no greater than 35 dB at least 80% of the time, as assessed by the ability to hear and understand normal conversation-level speech or, if necessary, as measured by an acoustic engineer. Children are allowed to make noise that doesn't exceed these limits. Controllable continuous noise, including playing of background music, is not allowed. To control excess voice noise coming from outside or inside the facility, teachers/caregivers model appropriate voice levels. The program installs noise abatement materials using fire-safe materials such as acoustical ceilings, wall coverings, partitions, or fabrics.[CFOC3 Std. 5.2.3.1]

5. **Food Safety:** (See Section 4: Nutrition, Food Handling, and Feeding.)

6. **Plastics:** This facility avoids using vinyl toys unless they are labeled polyvinylchloride (PVC) free, as well as other plastic items and toys unless they are labeled phthalate free and bisphenol A (BPA) free or ANSI certified.

   _____

   TITLE/NAME OF STAFF MEMBER

   checks and preferentially chooses any plastics for use in this facility with the recycle codes of 2, 4, or 5. Food and beverages are not heated in plastic containers or when covered with plastic wrap that touches the food. Plastic food containers, toys, feeding bottles, and spill-resistant drinking cups labeled without a recycle number or with the number 3, 6, or 7 are not used. Scratched plastic articles are thrown away.[CFOC3 Stds. 4.8.0, 5.2.9.9]

7. Mold:

_____
TITLE/NAME OF STAFF MEMBER

monitors humidity levels in the facility as indicated in Section 8.A.1.c.

_____
TITLE/NAME OF STAFF MEMBER

inspects and arranges drying and disinfection of all potentially moist surfaces of the facility indoors and outdoors to rid the premises of persistent moisture or excessive humidity that fosters mold growth.[CFOC3 Stds. 5.2.1.1, 5.2.1.6, 5.2.1.15, 6.2.4]

8. Furnishings and Equipment

a. **Foam:** Any item, including furniture, nap mats, and toys, with exposed foam is removed to avoid exposure to toxic flame retardants commonly found in foam.

b. **Particleboard:** This facility minimizes use of objects made with particleboard. Wall-to-wall carpeting installations are not allowed because they may put toxic chemicals into the air.

c. **Rugs/Carpeting:** Only rugs that can be laundered are permitted.

d. **Pressure-Treated Wood:** This facility _____ have any chromate copper arsenate (CCA)-
          DOES/DOES NOT

treated wood surfaces accessible to children (CCA pressure-treated wood). (Alternate: This facility has CCA pressure-treated wood, but it is coated with a penetrating sealer every 6 months.)[CFOC3 Std. 5.2.9.12]

e. **Carbon Monoxide Sources:** Indoor pollution from furnaces, kerosene and pellet stoves, fireplaces, gas-fired appliances such as generators, other gas-burning appliances such as stoves, idling vehicles near the building, and any other potential source of carbon monoxide are monitored by carbon monoxide alarms[CFOC3 Stds. 5.2.1.10, 5.2.1.11, 5.2.9.5] located

_____
LOCATION OF THE ALARMS.

Monthly,

_____
TITLE/NAME OF STAFF MEMBER

checks the alarms to be sure they function properly and that they are replaced every 5 years and documents the results in a file kept

_____
LOCATION OF THE FILE.

f. **Hot Surfaces:** Any hot surface such as a radiator/heater, hot water pipe, stove, or portable cooking equipment (eg, slow cooker, electric fry pan, toaster oven) that can be hotter than 120°F is made inaccessible to children with a guard or other protective device. An exception may be allowed for school-aged children using cooking equipment as intended by the manufacturer of the equipment with 1:1 supervision.[CFOC3 Std. 5.2.1.13]

9. Art Supplies and Sensory Materials

  a. **Approved Art Supplies:** This program uses only labeled, nontoxic art supplies with the Approved Product (AP) seal indicating they are approved by the Art & Creative Materials Institute.

  b. **Donated Articles:** Donated articles are not accepted unless they are labeled by their manufacturer and the label provides sufficient information for staff members to check and be sure they do not contain toxic substances.

  c. **Prohibited Materials:** No art materials that emit VOCs are used.[CFOC3 Stds. 5.2.9.7, 5.2.9.8]

  d. **Sensory Materials:** When children use sensory materials such as clay and homemade or commercial modeling compound (eg, Play-Doh),

  _____

  TITLE/NAME OF STAFF MEMBER

  verifies that the material is nontoxic. Children must wash their hands before and after handling the material. Teachers/caregivers clean and sanitize the surface and tools involved in this type of play before and after each use. The material is discarded after it is used by children who have cuts or sores or any sign of an infectious disease such as a runny nose.[CFOC3 Std. 5.2.9.8]

  e. **Sand and Similar Particulate Play Materials:** Sand must be clean and free of toxic materials or access by animals or insects, kept in containers that permit drainage so the sand can be washed, and have covers that staff members put over the sand when it is not being used.[CFOC3 Std. 6.2.4.1]

10. Plants:

  _____

  TITLE/NAME OF STAFF MEMBER

  is responsible for checking that all plants are not poisonous by reviewing the names of all plants indoors and in outdoor play areas with the local poison control center. Only plants known to be nonpoisonous that do not generate a lot of pollen in the air and do not drop small flowers or leaves are permitted anywhere inside or outside on the facility premises.[CFOC3 Std. 5.2.9.10]

  a. **Edible Plants:** Children are not allowed to put plants or edible parts of plants in their mouths unless the part of the plant to be mouthed has been washed and is suitable as food.

  b. **Poisonous Plants:** Any contact with a potentially poisonous plant requires an immediate call to Poison Help (1-800-222-1222) for instructions and notification of the family.

11. Sun Safety: This facility protects children and staff members from the harmful effects of ultraviolet (UV) radiation, using the following measures:

  a. **Protection From Injury From Exposure to the Sun:**

   i. The program arranges for shade and encourages use of shade in outdoor play areas and areas where children go for field trips. In addition to application of sunscreen as indicated on the product label, for outdoor play and field trips that occur between 10:00 am and 2:00 pm, children and teachers/caregivers must wear sun-protective clothing and/or be in shaded areas. Infants younger than 6 months are kept out of direct sunlight.[CFOC3 Std. 3.4.5.1]

   ii. To be outdoors in sunlight, all children are dressed in cool, comfortable, lightweight, tightly woven (sun-protective) clothing that covers the body but allows evaporation of sweat. They wear a wide-brimmed hat that shadows the eyes, ears, face, and neck.

   iii. Parents/legal guardians are asked to provide shatter-resistant sunglasses that block 99% to 100% of UV light for children to wear when exposed to the sun.

iv. Teachers/caregivers apply sunscreen of SPF 50 no less than 15 to 30 minutes prior to sun exposure on skin that is not protected by clothing.

_____

TITLE/NAME OF STAFF MEMBER

collects a signed authorization and instruction for use of sunscreen and how to apply it from parents/legal guardians. (See Appendix T: Sun Safety Permission Form.) This facility

_____

PURCHASES BULK SUPPLIES OF A SINGLE BRAND OF SUNSCREEN TO APPLY TO ALL CHILDREN WHOSE PARENTS/LEGAL GUARDIANS AUTHORIZE THIS BRAND, OR APPLY THE SPECIFIC SUNSCREEN PRODUCT THAT PARENTS/LEGAL GUARDIANS PROVIDE FOR THEIR CHILD.

Sunscreen is reapplied approximately every 2 hours if children continue to be exposed to sun.[CFOC3 Std. 3.4.5.1]

b. **Checking the UV Index:**

_____

TITLE/NAME OF STAFF MEMBER

checks the UV index provided by the EPA on the Internet at www.epa.gov/sunwise/uvindex.html or by listening to local news broadcasts to plan sun-safe activities for the locations where outdoor program activities occur.

12. Lead

a. **Lead Exposure From Building Surfaces:** The existing building and any previously constructed building that was on this site were built after 1978 when lead paint was no longer used. (Or, the building has been inspected by a qualified lead inspector and found free of lead paint; or, all painted woodwork is washed and inspected monthly by

_____

TITLE/NAME OF STAFF MEMBER

to be sure it is free of flaking, peeling, or chipped paint.)[CFOC3 Std. 5.2.9.13] The surfaces in and grounds around this facility, including all food preparation surfaces, have been determined free of lead hazard by

_____

METHODS OF CHECKING USED AND TYPE AND LOCATION OF DOCUMENTS ON FILE.

b. **Drinking Water:** The drinking water has been tested by

_____

METHODS OF CHECKING USED AND TYPE AND LOCATION OF DOCUMENTS ON FILE

and found to be free of lead hazard. Only cold water is used for drinking and cooking. The EPA recommends, "Anytime the water in a particular faucet has not been used for six hours or longer, 'flush' your cold-water pipes by running the water until it becomes as cold as it will get. This could take as little as five to thirty seconds if there has been recent heavy water use....Otherwise, it could take two minutes or longer. Your water utility will inform you if longer flushing times are needed to respond to local conditions."[2, CFOC3 Std. 5.2.6.3]

c. **Products that Might Contain Lead:** Although the regulations of the US Consumer Product Safety Commission (CPSC) make it illegal to sell toys that contain lead,

_____

TITLE/NAME OF STAFF MEMBER

checks the safety of our equipment and supplies with the CPSC list of items that have been recalled for lead or any other hazard. New purchases are checked at www.healthystuff.org to avoid those known to contain toxic chemicals. Products that might contain lead, such as imported ceramics and jewelry not certified lead free, are not allowed.[CFOC3 Std. 4.5.0.2]

d. **Prevention of Exposure to Harmful Substances in Soil on Shoes:** Soil-catching mats are outside and just inside each entry door from outside to the facility to help remove potentially harmful substances in outdoor dirt, such as lead.

13. **Soil and Play Area:** The environmental audit conducted for this facility for hazardous materials, including lead and pesticides on the grounds and in the soil and arsenic-treated wood equipment was conducted on

_____

DATE.

The result of the inspection includes the findings of the audit, any recommended corrective action, and what corrective action was taken.[CFOC3 Std. 5.1.1.5] The inspection report is on file in

_____

LOCATION OF FILED DOCUMENTATION.

14. **Mercury:** Mercury-containing thermometers or thermostats are not used in our facility. Mercury-containing compact fluorescent lights or bulbs are disposed of as required by our local hazardous waste processing facility.

15. **Asbestos and Fiberglass:** This facility was inspected for friable asbestos and fiberglass on

_____

DATE.

Any recommended remedial action is performed by a certified contractor.[CFOC3 Std. 5.2.9.6] The inspection report and actions taken are on file in

_____

LOCATION OF DOCUMENTATION OF THE INSPECTION AND CORRECTIVE ACTIONS.

16. **Radon:** This facility was tested for the presence of radon following the EPA protocol that required testing for more than 90 days with alpha-track or electret test devices.[CFOC3 Std. 5.2.9.4] The report of this test and any recommended remedial action is in

_____

LOCATION WHERE TEST DOCUMENT IS FILED.

17. **Recycling:** This facility recycles articles that are authorized for recycling by our solid waste service.

B. Hazard/Safety Checks and Corrective Actions

1. **Total Facility Hazard/Safety Checks:** Using adaptations of nationally recommended health and safety facility checklists or applicable state, tribal, or territory checklists,

---

TITLES/NAMES OF STAFF MEMBERS

perform and document the results of at least monthly inspections.

TITLE/NAME OF STAFF MEMBER

assigns responsibility for implementation and tracks dated corrective action plans. (See "ECELS Health and Safety Checklist with References" at www.ecels-healthychildcarepa.org/component/k2/item/255-ecels-health-and-safety-checklist-2011-references. This form is widely used. Each item is cross-referenced with *CFOC3* and the Environment Rating Scales, as well as Pennsylvania state child care regulations, which users could switch for their own state requirements.)*CFOC3* Stds. 5.7.0.2, 6.1.0.1, 6.1.0.2, 6.2.1.1–6.2.1.9, 6.2.5.1, 6.2.5.2

2. **Outdoor and Indoor Large-Muscle Play Areas**

   a. **Areas Used for Large-Muscle Play:** Our facility uses the following areas for indoor and outdoor large-muscle play:

   LOCATIONS OF AGE-SEPARATED AREAS USED FOR INDOOR OR OUTDOOR LARGE-MUSCLE PLAY ON FACILITY PREMISES AND ANYWHERE ELSE FOR ALL INFANTS, TODDLERS, AND PRESCHOOL- AND SCHOOL-AGED GROUPS SERVED.

   b. **Inspections of Play Areas and Equipment:**

   TITLE/NAME OF STAFF MEMBER

   makes daily inspections of play areas and equipment available for use indoors and outdoors. (See Appendix O: Daily and Monthly Playground Inspection and Maintenance.)

   TITLE/NAME OF STAFF MEMBER

   conducts monthly inspections to ensure that surfaces, spacing of activities, and any equipment used for large-muscle play meet the guidelines/standards of the CPSC and ASTM. (See Appendix O: Daily and Monthly Playground Inspection and Maintenance.)

3. **Toys:**

TITLE/NAME OF STAFF MEMBER

is responsible for checking that all toys meet the following requirements*CFOC3* Stds. 3.3.0.2, 5.3.1.4, 6.4.1.2:

   a. **Infants and Toddlers:**

      i. Each group of children in diapers has its own toys and does not share toys with other groups. Children in diapers have only washable toys. Any cloth toys for children who are still mouthing toys are used by only one child before being laundered and are laundered whenever heavily soiled.

ii.   All toys that are mouthed during the course of the day are set aside in an inaccessible container for cleaning before another child plays with the toy. Mouthed toys are thoroughly cleaned and sanitized. Toys may be washed and sanitized by hand or by washing in a dishwasher.

iii. Toys accessible to children younger than 3 years have no removable small parts, a diameter of less than 1¼ inches and a length of less than 2¼ inches (or a diameter of less than 1¾ inches if round or egg shaped), and are not small enough to fit completely in a child's mouth.

iv.   For children younger than 3 years, strings on toys are no longer than 12 inches. Straps are removed from hats/guitars or other articles accessible to children in this age group.

v.   No magnets, plastic bags, or Styrofoam objects are accessible to children younger than 3 years.

b.   **Preschool-aged Children:** Latex balloons are not accessible to children younger than 8 years.[CFOC3 Std. 6.4.1.5]

c.   **Cleaning of Toys:** All toys are cleaned at least weekly and whenever visibly soiled. Toys that develop sharp edges or loose parts, are rusty, are coated with lead paint, have breakable glass, or present risks of injury from common use are repaired or discarded.

4. **Documentation of Safety Inspections, Incidents, and Corrective Action Plans:** All safety inspection and incident reports, including corresponding corrective action plans, are reviewed by

---

TITLE/NAME OF STAFF MEMBER OR GROUP

at least quarterly to identify any further action needed and assign follow-up responsibility.

References

1.   US Environmental Protection Agency. *America's Children and the Environment*. 3rd ed. Washington, DC: US Environmental Protection Agency; 2013. EPA 240-R-13-001. http://www.epa.gov/ace/publications/ACE3_2013.pdf. Accessed August 28, 2013

2.   US Environmental Protection Agency. Basic information about lead in drinking water. http://water.epa.gov/drink/contaminants/basicinformation/lead.cfm. Accessed August 28, 2013

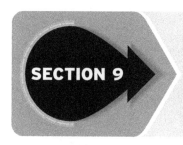

Transportation (Motor Vehicle, Bicycle/ Tricycle, or Other Wheeled Toys), Pedestrian Safety, and Field Trips

Rationale

Motor vehicle crashes and pedestrian injuries are the leading cause of death in children after infancy. Use of wheeled toys such as bicycles is a major cause of traumatic brain injury and limb fractures. Trips away from the facility bring children and staff into less familiar environments that may expose them to significant hazards.

Required Action/Who Is Responsible/How Communicated

A. Motor Vehicles and Drivers Used for Program Activities[CFOC3 Std. 9.2.5.1]

1. **Vehicle Type, Vehicle License, Driver License/Certification, and Insurance:** Vehicles are those that legally qualify as school buses or otherwise qualify for transport of children according to CFOC3.[CFOC3 Std. 6.5.3.1] Vehicles and drivers are licensed according to state law and insured for the type of transport being provided. Documentation of current licenses and insurance is on file in

_____

LOCATION.

_____

TITLE/NAME OF STAFF MEMBER

ensures that the facility has documentation that drivers meet all the requirements related to child abuse and criminal clearances and have current certification of satisfactory completion of training in pediatric first aid/cardiopulmonary resuscitation.

2. **Emergency Equipment and Supplies:** Vehicles are equipped with a first aid kit, emergency information for all children being transported, and a functioning cell phone, 2-way radio, or other mobile communication device. Someone in the vehicle knows how to call 911 and how to notify the facility and families of passengers and the driver. A backup vehicle is available at

_____

LOCATION

and can be dispatched immediately in case of an emergency. Drivers carry information with the quickest route to an emergency medical facility from any point from start to destination.[CFOC3 Std. 6.5.2.6]

3. **Vehicle Climate Control:** Vehicles are air-conditioned when providing fresh air through open windows does not reduce the temperature inside the vehicle below 82°F. Vehicles are heated when temperatures drop below 65°F and when children feel cold.[CFOC3 Std. 6.5.2.4]

4. **Prevention of Inappropriate Use:** Vehicles are locked when not in use. Weekly,

---

TITLE/NAME OF STAFF MEMBER

inspects all vehicles and passenger restraint systems used by the facility to be sure they are kept clean and safe (interior and exterior).

5. **Forms Carried in Vehicles:** Vehicles are equipped with a notebook containing a weekly safety checklist with corrections made, incident report forms, and a trip sheet to record destination, mileage, times of departure and return, and a list of passengers with their emergency contact and medical information.

6. **Driver Training:** Drivers receive instruction and demonstrate ability to implement the required safety procedures.

   a. **Instruction:** Local traffic safety professionals from

   ---

   POLICE OR OTHER GOVERNMENT SAFETY EXPERTS

   provide instruction for individuals who provide motor vehicle transportation for this facility. Documentation of this training for drivers is available in

   ---

   LOCATION OF DOCUMENTATION.

   b. **Required Safety Procedures:** Anyone involved in providing transportation of children for this facility must be oriented to and follow the specific requirements in these policies and detailed in supplemental procedure documents for

      i.   Use of safety restraints

      ii. Permissible drop-off and pickup sites and routines

      iii. How to check the vehicle before and after each trip for children who might be behind, under, or in the vehicle before and after each trip

      iv. Handling of emergency situations

      v.   Transportation of children with special needs specific to the accommodation required by the children with special needs to be transported by a driver

      vi. Responsibility for supervision of children assigned to others while traveling and acceptable child supervision roles that drivers may assume in unusual situations that involve the vehicle or passengers

B. Use of Motor Vehicles

1. Selection of Drivers:

TITLE/NAME OF STAFF MEMBER

ensures that drivers are selected following the human resources policies of the facility and have the qualifications and training detailed in *CFOC3*.[CFOC3 Stds. 6.5.1.1, 6.5.1.2] Anyone who drives children (other than his or her own children) on behalf of the facility must meet the requirements for drivers and vehicles.

2. **Emptying and Locking Vehicles:** All vehicles are locked when not in use.

TITLE/NAME OF STAFF MEMBER

does a face-to-name count of children before and after transporting to be sure all children are placed in the vehicle and none are left in an unattended vehicle.[CFOC3 Std. 6.5.2.4]

3. **Drop-off and Pickup:** The facility has and communicates to staff and parents/guardians a plan on file

---
LOCATION WHERE PLAN IS AVAILABLE

for safe, supervised drop-off and pickup points and pedestrian crosswalks in the vicinity of the facility. Drop-off and pickup are allowed only at the curbside of vehicles or at an off-street location protected from traffic.

TITLE/NAME OF STAFF MEMBERS

supervise drop-off, pickup, and loading of vehicles and make sure children are clear of the perimeter of all vehicles and properly buckled into their car seat restraints before any vehicle moves.

TITLE/NAME OF STAFF MEMBER

keeps an accurate attendance and time record of all children picked up and dropped off. The adult who is supervising the child stays with the child until the responsibility for that child has been accepted by the individual designated in advance to assume care for that child.[CFOC3 Std. 6.5.2.1]

4. **Child:Staff Ratios During Transport:** Child:staff ratios during transport are the same as those used for daily classroom/group activities. (See Section 2.A: Child:Staff Ratios, Group Size, and Staff Qualifications.) Drivers are not counted in the staff ratio and are not responsible for managing the behavior of children while driving. Drivers do not use alcohol for at least 12 hours before driving and do not use any drugs of any type that can impair driving skills.

5. **Number of People Transported:** The number of adults and children transported in the vehicle is limited to the manufacturer's stated capacity for the vehicle.

6. **Child Passenger Safety:** When children are in a vehicle that meets current standards for a school bus or public bus intended to transport children of the age of the passengers in it, the seat compartment or other restraint systems of that vehicle are used only for the size of children and in the way intended by the manufacturer, with seat belts if those are provided. When children are in any other type of vehicle, the manufacturer's recommendations for securing passengers are followed.[CFOC3 Std. 6.5.2.2]

    a. **Use of Seat Restraints:** For transportation provided or arranged by the program/facility, staff members secure each child in a car safety seat, booster seat, seat belt, or harness adjusted to fit the child and selected to be appropriate to the child's weight, age, and/or development according to state and federal laws (federal Motor Vehicle Safety Standard 213) and regulations as well as the manufacturer's instructions. Children are put in a shoulder/lap belt only when they reach 4 feet 9 inches tall and when, all the way back on the seat (with their hips where the back and horizontal portion of the seat meet), their knees bend to a 90-degree angle at the edge of the seat. Infants and toddlers ride rear-facing until they are 2 years of age or reach the upper limits of weight and height for their rear-facing seat. Children do not ride in the front passenger seat until they are at least 13 years old.[CFOC3 Std. 6.5.2.2]

b. **Car Seats That Belong to Individual Children:**

TITLE/NAME OF STAFF MEMBER

ensures that car seats provided by parents or by the program are labeled with the name and contact information of the child being transported at the time. This measure helps with proper identification and notification when a group of children is being transported and an accident occurs. Car seats that belong to individual children may be stored between arrival and departure in

---

LOCATION.

Monthly,

TITLE/NAME OF STAFF MEMBER

checks the recall list maintained by the National Highway Traffic Safety Administration (NHTSA) for car seats that cannot be used.

c. **Checking for Hot Metal Parts of Seat Restraints:** The staff members who are loading children check metal parts of the seat restraints to be sure they are not too hot to be against the child.

d. **Allowable Travel Times:** Travel plans include limiting transportation times for infants to minimize the time they are sedentary. Travel times for any child are limited to no more than 45 minutes, one way, on a daily basis.

e. **Activities for Children During Travel:** Teachers/caregivers interact with children who are awake while traveling by telling stories, singing songs, playing games, or talking about what the children see, especially traffic signs and lights. These activities are at a level that does not distract the driver.

7. **Field Trips:** Travel away from the facility is limited to walking excursions or those for which parents/legal guardians can drive their own children or the children are transported in a vehicle provided or arranged by the program/facility that is equipped with age-appropriate seat restraints for the children who are traveling in them. Each child wears identification with the child's name and the name and contact information of the child care program in a fashion that does not allow it to be easily read from a distance by a stranger. Staff members carry photographs and emergency contact information for each child. A parent/legal guardian must sign an informed consent for the specific trip for the child to go on that trip.

TITLE/NAME OF STAFF MEMBER

assigns children individually to a responsible adult. The responsible adults count the children assigned to them by matching faces to names at least every 15 minutes while on a field trip. The program does not assume responsibility for arrangements made by parents to have other parents transport their children.

8. **Wheelchair Transport:** For children who travel in wheelchairs, each wheelchair is installed in the vehicle with 4-point tie-downs in a forward-facing direction and a 3-point restraint system for the occupant separate from the wheelchair restraint. The tie-down system is placed through the wheelchair in the exact location specified by the manufacturer. Only wheelchairs that are labeled as suitable for use in transportation and vehicles equipped with a matching tie-down system are used in a vehicle. Children who need other functional adaptations for transportation are accommodated according to the written plan developed by the specialists who provide their specialized care.

9. **Prohibited Activities in Vehicles:** Leaving a child unattended; riding without a seat restraint; smoking at any time; playing of radios/CDs/other sound-making or media devices; earphones, earplugs, earbuds, or cell phones/texting devices except when the vehicle is parked or in an emergency; and eating or drinking in the vehicle are all prohibited.[CFOC3 Stds. 3.4.1.1, 6.5.2.5]

10. **Education About Child Passenger Safety**

    a. **Identification and Involvement of a Child Passenger Safety Trainer:**

    _____

    TITLE/NAME OF STAFF MEMBER

    identifies a source of qualified, specialized child passenger training by calling the NHTSA at 888/327-4236 or sending an e-mail inquiry using the e-mail message service on the NHTSA Web site at www.nhtsa.gov/Contact and then arranges for education of staff and parents/legal guardians about safe transport of children and safety measures related to transport of children in whatever vehicles the facility uses.

    b. **Teaching and Monitoring Child Passenger Safety:** Teachers/caregivers monitor and teach children about passenger safety inside and around the outside of the vehicle. Those who use a bus for transport are taught and monitored to be sure that they stay out of the 10-foot danger zone around the vehicle—the zone that is not visible to the driver.

11. **Seat Restraint Use by Families:**

    _____

    TITLE/NAME OF STAFF MEMBER

    reminds parents/legal guardians who do not provide or resist using age- and size-appropriate car seat restraints about the significant risk involved and any laws that require use of seat restraints for transport.[CFOC3 Std. 6.5.2.2]

12. **Route/Trip Planning:** All routes/trips are planned in advance, determining location of restrooms, sources of water, and location of emergency medical facilities.

13. **Oversight of Transportation Policies:**

    _____

    TITLE/NAME OF PROGRAM DIRECTOR/ADMINISTRATOR/SUPERVISOR

    spot-checks compliance with the transportation policies at least monthly.

C. Walking and Walking Trips

1. **Teaching and Modeling Pedestrian Safety:** Teachers/caregivers teach children about pedestrian safety by modeling and verbal reinforcement. Teachers/caregivers teach children to use crosswalks, corners as crossing points, sidewalks, and traffic signals when they are available within ¼ mile of crossing where vehicles travel and only after looking left, right, and left again, using their eyes to scan as they turn, like a flashlight.

2. **Keeping the Group of Children Together:** Teachers/caregivers keep toddlers and preschool-aged children together through use of a travel rope (a knotted rope stretched between 2 teachers/caregivers to which children hold on while they walk), by having an adult hold each child's hand, or by another means that keeps the children physically connected to an adult at all times. A designated adult supervises the children at the front of each group, and another adult supervises children at the back of each group.

3. **Identification of Safety Crosswalks, Drop-off/Pickup Locations, and Bike and Walking Routes:** In consultation with local police,

_____

TITLE/NAME OF STAFF MEMBER

designates and posts in a conspicuous place all the safe pedestrian crosswalks, drop-off and pickup points, and bike and walking routes around the facility.[CFOC3 Std. 5.1.6.1]

D. Biking, Riding, and Use of Wheeled Toys

School-aged children may bike along bicycle routes reviewed with the police and designated by the facility. Children older than 1 year must wear safety helmets when biking and using riding toys or wheeled equipment such as skateboards, in-line skates, and scooters. Helmets must be removed after finishing play for which helmets are required, before playing on other equipment.[CFOC3 Stds. 6.4.2.2, 6.4.2.3]

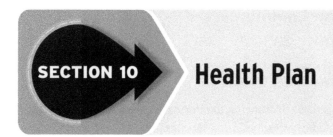

Rationale

Routine preventive health services for children and adults promote health and reduce diseases. Some diseases are detected that would otherwise become known at a later time, when the disease is more difficult to treat. Vaccines teach the body's immune system to resist infections and often prevent diseases from occurring at all. If the person gets the disease, it is milder than it would have been otherwise.

When children receive care from people other than their parents/legal guardians, everyone involved in the child's care should exchange information about the child and coordinate plans for the child's care. Teachers/caregivers, caregiving family members, and professionals who provide services for the child need to be briefed about what each knows and recommends. The child's usual source of health care (the *medical home*) is an especially important participant in reciprocal information sharing. Everyone needs parental/guardian permission to share confidential information about a child.

For staff members and volunteers, early education and child care programs should engage in reciprocal information sharing with health care professionals that is relevant to the worker's specific tasks. The primary health care professional of the paid or volunteer staff member needs this information to be able to address current and future job-related health concerns. Sharing this information enables the health care professional to suggest any accommodations the worker might need.

Checking and promoting the well-being of each person in the facility is essential to ensuring each person's ability to participate fully in a quality program. Adults need to be healthy to provide quality care. Children need to be healthy to fully participate in and benefit from the program. Teachers/caregivers need to know what accommodations children require. Administrators/directors need to know what special arrangements staff members with special needs require.

Practice of health-promoting behaviors in child care can have long-lasting benefits. For example, toothbrushing after meals and before bedtime with an age-appropriate amount of fluoride toothpaste prevents tooth decay by disrupting formation of plaque, strengthening tooth enamel, and teaching an effective preventive health habit.

Required Action/Who Is Responsible/How Communicated

A. Child and Staff Health Services

1. Child Health Assessment

a. **Routine Health Supervision:** The program must have documentation that each enrolled child is up to date with the schedule of nationally recommended health supervision services. The American Academy of Pediatrics (AAP) publishes the nationally recommended schedule, "Recommendations for Preventive Pediatric Health Care" (See Appendix D: Recommendations for Preventive Pediatric Health Care.)$^{CFOC3 \text{ Std.}}$ $^{3.1.2.1}$ The schedule specifies the ages at which children should receive routine screening assessments/tests, immunizations, and monitoring of chronic or acute illnesses. Parents/legal guardians must give documentation of the results of an age-appropriate health assessment to

_____

TITLE/NAME OF STAFF MEMBER

before the child begins to receive care. If a child has a pending appointment to receive the services, the program may allow attendance for

_____

6 WEEKS OR PROGRAM OR STATE REQUIREMENT, IF DIFFERENT

after the child starts receiving care. As long as documentation shows the results of an age-appropriate health assessment, a separate, extra health assessment for participation in the program is not necessary. Parents/legal guardians are responsible for making sure that their child receives routine health care on time and for giving

_____

TITLE/NAME OF STAFF MEMBER

a copy of the results of each of the child's subsequent health assessments after the initial assessment. Routine health supervision services should include

i. Reviewing the child's health history to identify health problems that may need special care, diet, sleep, and activity patterns; behavior and development; and any family health issues.

ii. Measuring growth and plotting of growth on standard charts from the World Health Organization, available at www.who.int/childgrowth/standards/en. After 24 months of age, growth assessment should include plotting body mass index on standardized charts available from the Centers for Disease Control and Prevention (CDC) at www.cdc.gov.

iii. Assessing development and social-emotional/behavioral health.

iv. Hearing screening.

v. Vision screening.

vi. Anemia screening.

vii. Evaluating oral health (and providing contact information for the child's dentist).

viii. Lead poisoning screening.

b. **Immunizations:** Each child must receive vaccines according to the current schedule published on the Web sites of the CDC (www.cdc.gov/vaccines) and AAP (www.aap.org/immunization) unless the child has a documented medical or other legally allowable exception.[CFOC3 Std. 7.2.0.1] Every year,

_____
TITLE/NAME OF STAFF MEMBER

checks these Web sites for updates to the recommended immunization schedules. This facility _____
                                                                                           WILL/WILL NOT
accept children who are under-immunized and, in addition, will follow state health department/child care regulating body regulations concerning attendance of children who are not immunized due to religious or medical reasons. Unimmunized or under-immunized children will be caught up as promptly as possible. Any who have exemptions from the requirement for up-to-date vaccines to participate in the program will be excluded during outbreaks of vaccine-preventable illness as directed by the state health department. (Optional: The parent of a child whose immunizations are not kept up to date and does not qualify for an exemption from receipt of required vaccines will be given the opportunity to review and sign the Refusal to Vaccinate form or be dismissed after 3 written reminders to the parent or legal guardian over a 3-month period. See Appendix E: Refusal to Vaccinate.) Staff members will encourage every family to obtain annual influenza vaccine for themselves and their children as directed by the AAP.

c. **Sharing of Pertinent Health Information:** With consent from the child's parent/legal guardian,

_____
TITLE/NAME OF STAFF MEMBER

shares health information necessary to the care of the child with health and education professionals involved with the child's care.[CFOC3 Std. 3.1.2.1]

d. **Daily Health Check:** Each day, the staff member who first assumes responsibility from the family for the care of a child performs and documents a health check. This daily health check includes a friendly greeting of the child and family member, asking the child and family member about the child's and family's well-being since the child was last in the facility, while observing the child for signs of obvious ill health. (See Appendix M: Instructions for Daily Health Check.) Based on the results of this interaction,

_____
TITLE/NAME OF STAFF MEMBER

determines whether those who are ill or injured can or cannot have their needs and those of the other children met, and if the child can participate in the program that day. If the child can stay but needs special care, the staff member makes a plan with the family for the time the child will be in the facility, verifying a method of easy contact with the parent/legal guardian during the day.[CFOC3 Stds. 3.1.1]

e. **Clarification of Health Concerns:** Questions raised by staff members at this program about the child's health will be directed by

_____
TITLE/NAME OF STAFF MEMBER

to the family or (with permission of parents/legal guardians) to the child's health care professional for explanation and implications for child care.

2. Adult Health Assessment^{CFOC3 Std. 1.7.0.1}

a. **Occupational Health:** Workers in this facility are informed by

_____

TITLE/NAME OF STAFF MEMBER

about special health concerns associated with their work roles. (See Appendix V: Major Occupational Health Hazards.) Risks related to infectious diseases include^{CFOC3 Stds. 1.7.0.4, 1.7.0.5, CFOC3 Appendix B}:

   i.   Exposure to infectious diseases

   ii. Falls

   iii. Musculoskeletal injuries related to lifting, squatting, and using child-sized furniture

   iv. Need for frequent hand hygiene

   v.   Use of cleaning, sanitizing, and disinfecting chemicals

   vi. Stress related to compensation and benefits, high expectations for performance, and little break/sick/personal time

   vii. Special health concerns for pregnant teachers/caregivers from infections and activities that can affect the outcome of their pregnancy

b. **Preemployment Health Appraisal:** All paid and volunteer staff members must have a health appraisal before their first involvement in child care work. The appraisal should identify any accommodations required for the staff person to carry out assigned duties per that person's job description. (See Section 16.B: Staff Health Assessment and Appendix W: Child Care Staff Health Assessment.) The staff health appraisal must include

   i.   Health history.

   ii. Physical examination.

   iii. Dental examination.

   iv. Vision and hearing screening.

   v.   Results and appropriate follow-up of tuberculosis (TB) screening using the tuberculin skin test or interferon-gamma release assay once on entry into the child care field with subsequent TB screening as determined by a history of high risk for TB thereafter (eg, foreign born, history of homelessness, HIV infected, contact with a prison population or someone with active TB).

   vi. Review and certification of up-to-date immune status per the current adult immunization schedule on the CDC Web site at www.cdc.gov/vaccines. Any staff person who is not up to date with current recommended vaccines will be reminded that this is a job-related requirement. Unless an under-immunized employee or volunteer person has a medical exemption for a specific type of vaccine, failure to obtain the vaccines recommended by the CDC is grounds for termination.

c. **Release to Return to Work After an Illness or Injury:** Staff members and volunteers must have their health care professional's release to return to work when they have a condition or an illness that may affect their ability to do their job, require accommodations to perform the tasks specified in their job descriptions, have a job-related injury, or have worker's compensation issues that put the facility at risk related to the health problem.^{CFOC3 Std. 1.7.0.3}

d. Daily Oversight of Staff Health:

_____

TITLE/NAME OF STAFF MEMBER

is responsible for observing all adults in the facility (staff members, volunteers, visitors) for signs of obvious ill health and directing those who are ill or injured to go home. Staff members and volunteers who are ill or injured (at the facility or elsewhere) report their condition immediately to their supervisor, who arranges for a substitute. [CFOC3 Std. 1.7.0.2]

3. Tracking and Updating Immunizations and Checkup Records:

_____

TITLE/NAME OF STAFF MEMBER

checks the facility's records to be sure each child's and each adult's immunization and other routine health supervision services are current

_____

FREQUENCY OF CHECKING (AT LEAST ANNUALLY; MORE OFTEN FOR YOUNGER CHILDREN).

_____

TITLE/NAME OF STAFF MEMBER

reminds parents/legal guardians and staff members to provide documentation of health assessments and provides reminders about when these assessments are overdue, due, or due soon. Staff members who refuse nationally recommended vaccines will be

_____

SELECT WHETHER STAFF WILL BE REQUIRED TO REVIEW, ACCEPT, AND SIGN THE REFUSAL TO VACCINATE FORM OR WILL BE SUSPENDED UNTIL THE VACCINES ARE RECEIVED. (SEE APPENDIX E: REFUSAL TO VACCINATE.)

B. Oral Health [CFOC3 Stds. 3.1.5.1–3.1.5.3, 5.5.0.1, 9.2.3.14]

1. **Food Choices:** This facility serves foods and beverages that are low in sugar, such as drinking water, with a preference for protein-, calcium-, and vitamin-rich foods such as milk, cheese, eggs, and fresh fruit and vegetables—foods that are good for nutrition and oral health.

2. **Pacifiers and Teething Rings:** Pacifiers and teething rings are used only by the child to whom the pacifier/teething ring belongs. Pacifiers may only be used in the child's crib for sleeping. Pacifiers and teething rings are cleaned when soiled and then cleaned and sanitized at the end of the day. Pacifiers that are damaged, have attachments, or are clipped, pinned, or tied to the child are not allowed.

3. **Bottles and No-Spill Cups:** Devices for children who cannot yet drink from a regular cup are used only during meals and snacks and while the child is held or seated. Children are weaned from the bottle or no-spill cup to drink from a regular cup as soon as the child shows interest and learns to do so. (See also Section 4: Nutrition, Food Handling, and Feeding.)

4. **Oral Hygiene:** As soon as a child's first tooth erupts, teachers/caregivers start oral hygiene with a soft toothbrush. Oral hygiene is a daily curricular activity for all children who have teeth.

  a. **Toothbrushing Procedure**
   i.   After performing hand hygiene, teachers/caregivers prepare a disposable paper cup by putting the portion of fluoride-containing toothpaste on the edge of the cup and provide each child with the child's individually assigned, clean toothbrush. Children who are ready to learn to swish and spit may have a small amount of water in the cup.

   ii.   The portion of fluoride-containing toothpaste for children younger than 2 years is a smear and for children older than 2 years is a small pea-sized amount.^CFOC3 Std. 3.1.5.1

   iii. For toothbrushing, children are seated at a table or stand at a sink that is not used for toileting or diapering. They are not allowed to walk around with or share their toothbrushes.

   iv.   The teachers/caregivers demonstrate toothbrushing to the children and assist a different child in the group each day so that each child learns how to properly brush. Wearing disposable gloves while assisting with toothbrushing is recommended. Because a longer duration of brushing leads to more plaque removal, the teachers/caregivers encourage children to brush for 2 minutes.

   v.   After brushing, children who are ready to learn to swish and spit and are not brushing their teeth at a sink are encouraged to use the water in the cup and spit the water back into the cup.

   vi.   After brushing, the teachers/caregivers rinse toothbrushes individually in running water and store them to dry so their bristles are up and do not touch any other surface. Paper cups are discarded in the trash.

   vii. Children and teachers/caregivers perform hand hygiene after toothbrushing.

   viii. _____
         FAMILIES OR THE PROGRAM

         provide a new toothbrush, labeled with the child's name, every 3 to 4 months or sooner if the bristles become frayed or the toothbrush becomes contaminated.^CFOC3 Std. 3.1.5.2

  b. **Water Rinsing After Eating:** When toothbrushing is not performed after eating, children are given a drink of water to rinse the food off their teeth.

5. **Fluoride in Drinking Water:** The drinking water at this facility _____ fluoride at the
   HAS/DOES NOT HAVE
   level recommended for better oral health. Drinking water with fluoride in combination with fluoride toothpaste prevents tooth decay.

6. **Dentist for Each Child:** Parents/legal guardians identify a dentist who cares for their child's teeth.

   _____
   TITLE/NAME OF STAFF MEMBER

   has lists of dentists in the community for families to use if they have not already found a dentist for their child.

7. **Tooth Decay and Dental Emergencies:** When opportunities arise for staff members to look at a child's teeth, especially behind the front teeth and under the lips, staff members note signs of tooth decay or injury such as discoloration of the teeth or patchy appearance of tooth color. Any concern is reported to the child's parents/legal guardians with a request to take the child to a dentist for evaluation of the observations. In the event of a dental emergency,

_____

TITLE/NAME OF STAFF MEMBER

immediately contacts the parents/legal guardians and the child's dentist or

_____

NAME OF DENTIST WHO ADVISES THE PROGRAM

for guidance.

8. **Oral Health Education:** Teachers/caregivers include activities about oral health in the curriculum.$^{CFOC3 \text{ Std. } 3.1.5.3}$

_____

TITLE/NAME OF STAFF MEMBER

arranges for dental health professionals to come to the facility to teach about oral health at least

_____

FREQUENCY OF VISITS.

C. Hazard/Safety Checks and Corrective Actions

See Section 8.B: Hazard/Safety Checks and Corrective Actions.

D. Obesity Prevention

See sections 4: Nutrition, Food Handling, and Feeding and 5: Physical Activity and Screen Time.

E. Children With Special Needs and Disabilities

See also sections 1.A: Admission; 2.A: Child:Staff Ratios, Group Size, and Staff Qualifications; and 4.F: Feeding of Children With Special Nutritional Needs.

1. **Care Plan**$^{CFOC3 \text{ Stds. } 3.5.0.1, 8.4.0.1}$: Children and adults who participate in the program and who require special adaptations or accommodations not required by typically developing children or other adults involved with the program must have a care plan that addresses routines and emergencies appropriate for that child. The care plan is completed by the individual's health care professionals and specialists with parents/legal guardians and

_____

TITLE/NAME OF STAFF MEMBER

with input from the program's health consultant, to determine the steps required to accommodate the person's needs. For children who are eligible for early intervention services, the care plan can be the Individual

Family Service Plan or Individual Education Plan developed with the assistance of the child's case manager for developmental disability services as required by the Individuals with Disabilities Education Act. In such situations, the coordinator for the child care program is

_____

TITLE/NAME OF STAFF MEMBER.

The care plan must be reviewed and updated as necessary each time the individual has a follow-up visit with a health care professional or specialist and no less than every 6 months. (See Appendix G: Special Care Plan Forms for 3 forms: "Care Plan for a Child With Special Needs in Child Care," "Behavioral Data Collection Sheet," and "Special Care Plan for a Child With Behavior Concerns," and see Appendix H: How to Use Special Care Plans.)

2. **Orientation and Training of Staff Members:** Individuals who are involved with children or coworkers with special needs are oriented and provided information to understand and meet the special needs. The orientation and education must be accomplished before the individual with special needs participates in the program. A care plan provided by the individual's primary health care professional or specialist informs arrangements for this orientation and training.[CFOC3 Std.1.4.2.2] Topics to address are any special handling, diet/feeding, medication, toileting issues, special treatments, adaptive equipment, abilities and limitations, recognition and response to emergencies, transport requirements, and methods of communication to use when clarification of the care plan is required.

3. **Specific Conditions** (See *Managing Chronic Health Needs in Child Care and Schools: A Quick Reference Guide* from the AAP for more detailed information about the following 2 most common health conditions and other special needs.)[1]

   a. **Food Allergy**[CFOC3 Std. 4.2.0.10]: In addition to following the instructions on the individual's care plan, the staff members involved in any way with the person with a food allergy will be taught and practice administering any prescribed medications that the allergic person might require in the event of an allergic reaction. To prevent inadvertent exposure of the person with a food allergy to the problem food, any food brought to the center is screened to be sure it does not contain any ingredients that require measures to prevent exposure of anyone in the facility who has a food allergy. With the consent of the parents/legal guardians of a child who has a food allergy,

   _____

   TITLE/NAME OF STAFF MEMBER

   posts the person's name, an easily recognized photo, and a list of that person's food allergies in every room in the facility ever occupied by that person to be sure that no visitor or substitute exposes the child to the offending food. Someone who has received instruction about how to follow the care plan will accompany the person who has the food allergy and bring emergency medications (eg, EpiPen) that may be required by that person on any field trip or excursion away from the posted areas.

   b. **Other Allergies and Asthma:** Every effort should be made to provide a way for someone with allergies or asthma to participate in all program activities by modifying the environment, using preventive medicine, wearing protective clothing, or using other measures that prevent the problem from occurring rather than avoiding the activity altogether. As for food allergy, for allergies to other substances, the program will, with the consent of the parent/legal guardian of the child or of the adult with the allergy, post an alert in the area occupied by such individuals. Children and adults with asthma will have an Asthma Action Plan in addition to the emergency information form in Appendix I. (Free copies of the Asthma Action Plan are available at www.nhlbi.nih.gov/health/public/lung/asthma/asthma_actplan.htm.) The care plan and emergency medication will accompany the child with asthma when off-site.

c. **Developmental/Behavioral Disabilities:** For children with developmental or behavioral concerns, the program staff and the child's parents/legal guardians complete the Behavioral Data Collection Sheet to describe the teacher's/caregiver's observations of the child. Parents/legal guardians take this form and a copy of the Special Care Plan for a Child With Behavioral Concerns form to their child's health care professional. Parents/legal guardians ask the child's health care professionals to complete the Special Care Plan and return the completed form to the child's teacher/caregiver. Staff members use the information to coordinate the child's care with the care the family provides at home. (See Section 10.E.1: Care Plan and www.ecels-healthychildcarepa.org/tools/forms for the checklist.)

F. Medication Administration^{CFOC3} Stds. 3.6.3.1, 9.4.2.6

1. Acceptable Requests for Medication Administration

a. **Limitation of Situations That Require Medication Administration by Program Staff Members:** Because administration of medication poses an extra burden for staff and having medication in the facility is a safety hazard, medication administration is limited to situations for which an agreement to give medicine outside child care hours cannot be made. Whenever possible, the first dose of medication should be given at home to see if the child has any type of reaction. Parents/legal guardians may administer medication to their own child during the child care day.

b. **Requirement for an Instruction or Prescription From a Licensed Health Care Professional:** Medication administration at this facility is limited to prescription or nonprescription (over-the-counter) medications ordered by a prescribing health care professional for a specific child and accompanied by written consent of the parent/legal guardian. The written order of the health professional must specify the medical reason for the medication, name of the medication, dose, route, when (ie, part of the day), for how long the medication is required (ie, number of days), and any reactions or side effects that might occur. Medications must be in their original pharmacy- or manufacturer-supplied container with a label that includes the child's name, date the medication was issued and when it expires, prescriber's name, dose/instructions, pharmacy name and phone number, and relevant warnings. Homemade or folk remedies are not accepted.

c. **Nonprescription Sunscreens, Diaper Creams, and Insect Repellents:** These products require written parent/legal guardian consent but do not require a written order from a health care professional. (See consent forms for sunscreen and insect repellents at www.ucsfchildcarehealth.org/pdfs/forms/Sunscr_SunSm.pdf and www.ucsfchildcarehealth.org/pdfs/forms/insectrepen.pdf, respectively.)

2. Symptom-Triggered Medication Administration: A licensed prescribing health care professional may state that a certain medication may be given for a recurring problem, emergency situation, or chronic condition. The instructions should include the child's name, name of the medication, dose of the medication, route, how often the medication may be given, conditions for use, and any precautions to follow. Any medication with instructions that state that the medication may be used whenever needed must be reviewed and renewed by the prescribing licensed health care professional at least annually. Standing orders for medication (ie, orders written in advance by a health care professional that describe the procedure to follow in defined situations) can be implemented only if the instructions for administration of the medication are clearly defined in the child's special care plan. An example of standing orders is a child who wheezes with vigorous exercise who may take one dose of asthma medicine before vigorous active (large-muscle) play. A child with a known serious allergic reaction to a specific substance who develops symptoms after exposure to that substance may receive epinephrine from a staff member who has received training in how to use an auto-injection device prescribed for that child (eg, EpiPen).

3. Staff Members Authorized to Give Medication in This Facility:

_____

TITLE/NAME OF STAFF MEMBERS

are the only people at this facility authorized to give medication. They have received training that includes the content provided in the Healthy Futures medication administration workshop curriculum or e-learning self-learning module provided by the AAP at www.healthychildcare.org/HealthyFutures.html and have demonstrated to a licensed health care professional the skills required to administer medication. (See the Medication Administration Observation Checklist at www.ecels-healthychildcarepa.org/tools/checklists.)

4. Storage of Medications: Medications are kept at the temperature recommended for that type of medication in a sturdy, child-resistant, closed container away from food or chemicals. The storage arrangement is inaccessible to children and prevents spillage.

5. Expired Medications: Medication is not used beyond the date of expiration on the container or beyond any expiration of the instructions provided by the physician or other person legally permitted to prescribe medication.

6. Documentation of Medication Administration:

_____

TITLE/NAME OF STAFF MEMBER

checks for the required information on the medication container and any accompanying instructions before accepting the medication. Medication is then stored properly and arrangements are made to administer and document the administration of each dose given as required. (See Appendix X: Medication Administration Packet.)

7. Medication Errors and Reactions to Medications

a. **Preventing Medication Errors:** Errors are prevented by checking and documenting the following 5 items each time medication is given:

    i.   Right child

    ii. Right medicine

    iii. Right dose

    iv. Right time

    v.   Right route of administration

b. **When a medication error occurs,**

_____

TITLE/NAME OF STAFF MEMBER

contacts the regional poison control center and the child's parents immediately. The error and what was done to handle it is documented in the child's record at the facility.

8. Medication Incidents: These incidents (eg, spitting out medication, spilling medication, a reaction to medication) are documented in the medication record for the child.

G. Health Education^{CFOC3} Stds. 2.4

1. **Topics:** Health education about physical, oral, mental, nutritional, and social health is part of the curriculum for staff, families, and children.

2. **Health Education Methods**

   a. **Developmentally Appropriate Teaching:** Teachers/caregivers use modeling and other types of developmentally appropriate instruction to teach children about health and safety.

   b. **Involving Community Professionals:** For preschool- and school-aged children, families, and staff members, instruction may include visits to community facilities or visits to the facility by health educators and health and safety professionals. Special projects related to the topic are sometimes arranged.

   _____
   TITLE/NAME OF STAFF MEMBER

   invites involvement in teaching health and safety topics from health educators, health care professionals, and community safety instructors from community hospitals, children's hospitals, voluntary health organizations, public health and public safety agencies, health/mental health/education consultants, local police, drug and alcohol programs, medical/oral health/nursing/mental health professionals and organizations, environmental health experts, other health agencies, and local colleges and universities.

   c. **Health Education Topics:** Topics taught include but are not limited to body functions and awareness, importance of routine preventive health care, diversity, personal social skills and expression of feelings, self-esteem, stress and conflict management, fitness/physical activity and indoor and outdoor play, nutrition, oral hygiene, early brain development, child development, prevention and control of infectious diseases, safety in the environment and personal behavior, first aid, emergency preparedness, rest and sleep, safe sleep for infants, management of chronic disease, and community resources.

3. **Calendar-Focused Health Education:**

   _____
   TITLE/NAME OF STAFF MEMBER

   asks local health agencies to identify upcoming celebrations of special health topics to coordinate planning for education in the facility with community activities on topics such as Child Passenger Safety Week, Children's Dental Health Month, American Heart Month, Week of the Young Child, and Fire Prevention Month. (See CFOC3 health education standards and standards about specific topics for contacts that may provide materials and suggested activities.)

4. **Notification of Families About Sensitive Topics:**

   _____
   TITLE/NAME OF STAFF MEMBER

   notifies parents/legal guardians if sensitive topic areas are included in the health education plan. Parents/legal guardians must respond to such notices with a written note if they do not want their child to be involved in activities related to a specific topic.

Reference

1. American Academy of Pediatrics. *Managing Chronic Health Needs in Child Care and Schools: A Quick Reference Guide.* Donoghue EA, Kraft CA, eds. Elk Grove Village, IL: American Academy of Pediatrics; 2010

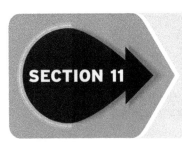
Care of Children and Staff Members Who Are Acutely Ill or Injured*CFOC3* Stds. 1.7.0.3, 3.6.1, 3.6.2.2–3.6.2.10, 7.3.11.1

Rationale

Infectious diseases and injuries are common occurrences among children and staff members who care for them. Policies must clearly state the procedures to follow to make decisions about when to exclude, when attendance is permitted, and when those who have been excluded may return. The care of children who are mildly ill in group care settings is an inevitable reality. During the winter, many children have a common respiratory illness (cold) at any one time and do not need to be excluded from the program unless their condition meets the exclusion criteria specified in these policies.

Required Action/Who Is Responsible/How Communicated

A. Admission and Exclusion

1. **Sharing Information:** All families are expected to openly share information about their child's behavior, symptoms, or exposure to illness. Families must have a backup plan for care of their children when the child is unable to be in the facility due to illness or injury. Staff members are expected to tell

   _____
   TITLE/NAME OF STAFF MEMBER

   about any symptoms, illness, or exposure to illness they experience themselves.

2. **Situations That Require a Note From a Health Care Professional:** A note from the child's or staff member's primary health care professional is necessary only when staff members need advice about any special care required by the child or staff member or if the child's or staff member's condition poses a health risk to others. Staff members rely on the family's description of the child's behavior or symptoms to determine when a child is well enough to return after an illness or injury.

3. **Authority for Decision to Admit or Exclude for Acute Illness:** Acute illness or injury is a temporary, short-term, usually infectious disease or injury.

   _____
   TITLE/NAME OF STAFF MEMBER WITH FINAL DECISION AUTHORITY

   decides about inclusion/exclusion, taking into account the current staffing situation and what is known about the illness or injury. The decision is informed by what the family and the child's teachers/caregivers share about the child's condition, current references, and findings of the daily health check procedure if the child is brought to the facility ill or injured or becomes ill or injured while in attendance. For staff members who are ill, the decision is made as for children except that the staff member who is ill or injured shares information about the condition with

   _____
   TITLE/NAME OF STAFF MEMBER

   who has final decision authority. The decision to exclude a child or staff member takes into account whether there are adequate facilities and staff members available to meet the needs of the person who is ill or injured and the other people at the facility at the time.

4. Criteria for Excluding Children Who Are Acutely Ill or Injured

a. **Ability to Participate:** The child's condition prevents the child from participating comfortably in activities that the facility routinely offers for well children or children who are mildly ill or injured.

b. **Need for More Care:** The condition requires more care than teachers/caregivers can provide without compromising the needs of the other children in the group.

c. **Risk to Others:** Keeping the child in care poses an increased risk to the child or other children or adults with whom the child comes in contact as defined in *Managing Infectious Diseases in Child Care and Schools.*[1]

5. Criteria for Excluding Staff Members Who Are Acutely ill or Injured: A staff member is excluded for illness or injury if the staff member cannot competently perform the duties as required by that staff member's job description or if the condition poses a risk to others in the facility.

6. Permitted Attendance and Care for Mild Illness: The following conditions or symptoms do not require exclusion:

- Common colds, runny noses (regardless of color or consistency of nasal discharge).
- A cough not associated with an infectious disease (eg, pertussis/whooping cough) or a fever (temperature of 100°F axillary/in an armpit, 101°F orally, 102°F rectally or equivalent reading with another type of thermometer). Rectal temperature taking requires specialized training and caution about possible concerns of child abuse.
- Watery yellow or white discharge or crusting eye discharge without fever, eye pain, or eyelid redness.
- Yellow or white eye drainage that is not associated with pink or red conjunctiva (ie, whites of the eyes).
- Pinkeye (bacterial conjunctivitis) indicated by pink or red conjunctiva with white or yellow eye mucous drainage and matted eyelids after sleep. Parents/guardians of children and staff members with conjunctivitis should seek and follow the advice about this condition provided by a primary care professional. If 2 unrelated children in the same program have conjunctivitis, the organism causing the conjunctivitis may have a higher risk of transmission and a child health care professional should be consulted.
- Fever without any signs or symptoms of illness in children who are older than 4 months regardless of whether acetaminophen or ibuprofen was given. Temperature above 100°F (37.8°C) axillary (armpit), 101°F (38.3°C) orally, 102°F (38.9°C) rectally, or measured by an equivalent method is a fever, an indication of the body's response to something. Body temperature can be elevated by overheating caused by overdressing or a hot environment, reactions to medications, and response to infection. If a child is behaving normally but has a body temperature above the thresholds indicated, the child should be monitored but does not need to be excluded for fever alone. Infants younger than 4 months with fever should be evaluated by a medical professional; infants younger than 2 months suspected to have an elevated body temperature should get medical attention immediately, within an hour if possible.
- Rash without fever and behavioral changes.
- Lice or nits (exclusion for treatment of an active lice infestation may be delayed until the end of the day).
- Ringworm (exclusion for treatment may be delayed until the end of the day).
- Molluscum contagiosum (do not require exclusion or covering of lesions).
- Thrush (ie, white spots or patches in the mouth or on the cheeks or gums).
- Fifth disease (slapped cheek disease, parvovirus B19) once the rash has appeared.
- Methicillin-resistant *Staphylococcus aureus* (MRSA) without an infection or illness that would otherwise require exclusion. Known MRSA carriers or colonized individuals should not be excluded.
- Cytomegalovirus infection.
- Chronic hepatitis B infection.
- HIV infection.

- Children and adults who had diarrhea and are now able to confine their stool to the toilet or diaper may return to care. For some infectious organisms, exclusion is required until certain guidelines have been met. These agents are not common, and teachers/caregivers usually do not know the cause of most cases of diarrhea.
- Children with chronic infectious conditions that can be accommodated in the program according to the legal requirement of federal law in the Americans with Disabilities Act. The act requires that child care programs make reasonable accommodations for children with disabilities and/or chronic illnesses, considering each child individually.

7. **State Regulations That Apply to Exclusion:** Our state's regulations require exclusion for the following conditions:

_____

CHECK SPECIFIC STATE REGULATIONS THAT MAY NOT CORRESPOND WITH CURRENT NATIONAL STANDARDS ON WHICH THIS POLICY IS BASED. STATE REGULATIONS ARE THE LEGAL FLOOR OF OPERATION AND MUST BE FOLLOWED.

B. Procedure for Management of Short-term Illness: If a child appears mildly ill but is staying for the day

1. **Complete an Admission Symptom Record:** The child's teacher/caregiver completes a symptom record to document date, time, and symptoms of illness. (See Appendix Y: Symptom Record.)

2. **Develop a Care Plan:** The teachers/caregivers and parent/legal guardian discuss treatment and develop a plan for the child's care. If the teachers/caregivers have questions or do not understand instructions provided by the health care professional for care of the child,

_____
TITLE/NAME OF STAFF MEMBER

will contact the child's health care professional with consent of the parent/legal guardian.

3. **Complete a Symptom Record:** The child's teachers/caregivers complete another symptom record during the period the child is in care and give a copy of this symptom record to the parent/legal guardian when the child leaves the program for the day.

4. **Increasing Symptoms While in Child Care:** If a child who was well at drop-off time becomes sick or a mildly ill child becomes sicker during the time the child is in care, the procedure is as follows:

   a. **Conditions That Require Medical Attention Right Away:** If the illness is one of those on the list of conditions that require medical attention right away, the child's teacher/caregiver notifies

_____
TITLE/NAME OF STAFF MEMBER

to call 911 and the parent/legal guardian, makes the child comfortable, and completes the symptom record form. (See Appendix Z: Situations That Require Medical Attention Right Away.)

   b. **Decision-maker About Inclusion/Exclusion:**

_____
TITLE/NAME OF STAFF MEMBER

determines whether the child may remain in the program or is too ill to stay.

c. **Contacting the Parent/Legal Guardian:** Whether the decision is to allow the child to stay or leave the facility,

---
TITLE/NAME OF STAFF MEMBER

calls the parent/legal guardian to discuss the symptoms and how the facility plans to manage the situation.

d. **Management of Symptoms for an Ill Child in the Facility:** The teachers/caregivers manage the child's symptoms until the child is transferred to the care of the parent/legal guardian or a previously authorized emergency contact person. The teachers/caregivers record the management on the symptom record.

e. **Obtaining Health Professional Advice:** If the facility needs the advice of a health care professional,

---
TITLE/NAME OF STAFF MEMBER

contacts the local or state health department or, with consent of the parent/legal guardian, the child's primary health care professional for advice.

f. **Arranging Pickup:** If the child is too ill to stay in child care, the facility asks the parent/legal guardian or a previously authorized emergency contact person to pick up the child as soon as possible. Until the child is picked up, the facility provides the child with a familiar teacher/caregiver to care for the child in a place where the child can rest.

g. **Use of the Symptom Record:** In addition to noting the child's symptoms on the group attendance record,

---
TITLE/NAME OF STAFF MEMBER

will place a copy of the symptom record in the child's file and give a copy of the symptom record to the parent/legal guardian. The staff member who greets the parent/legal guardian at pickup encourages the parent/legal guardian to use the symptom record to continue the child's care and, if necessary, to provide the information to the child's health care professional for management of the child's illness.

h. **Location of Children Who Are Being Excluded for Illness While Waiting for Pickup:** A child with a potentially contagious illness that requires that the child be sent home from child care will receive care in a location where the child can be separated from other children by at least 3 feet until the child leaves the facility. This arrangement may be in the child's usual care setting with extra attention to hygiene and sanitation. The location will avoid exposure of people not previously in close contact with the child and be where the child's needs can be met under close supervision.

i. **Medication:** See Section 10.F: Medication Administration.

C. Reporting Requirements

1. **Reportable Diseases:** Some communicable diseases must be reported to public health authorities so that required control measures can be used.

TITLE/NAME OF STAFF MEMBER

obtains an updated list of reportable diseases from local or state health authorities annually and shares a copy of this list with each parent/legal guardian at the time of enrollment.

2. **Responsibility for Reporting Illness:** Each September,

_____

TITLE/NAME OF STAFF MEMBER

reminds families and staff members to notify

_____

TITLE/NAME OF STAFF MEMBER

within 24 hours after a child, staff member, or member of the child's or staff member's immediate household develops a known or suspected communicable disease and if the condition is a reportable communicable disease.

3. **Notification of the Public Health Department:** While respecting the legal boundaries of confidentiality of medical information,

_____

TITLE/NAME OF STAFF MEMBER

notifies the appropriate public health department authority about any suspected or confirmed reportable disease among the children, staff members, or family members of the children and staff members and then follows the advice of the health department about additional notifications that may be necessary. (See Appendix AA: Sample Letter to Families About Exposure to Communicable Disease.) The telephone number of the responsible local or state public health authority to whom to report communicable diseases is

_____

PHONE NUMBER.

D. Obtaining Immediate Medical Help

See Section 13.F: Emergency and Evacuation Plan, Drills, and Closings.

E. Outbreaks of Disease

1. **Reporting Outbreaks of Infectious Disease:** If more than 2 cases of an infectious disease other than the common cold occur in a group of children/staff members who are in close contact with one another,

_____

TITLE/NAME OF STAFF MEMBER

calls the local/state public health department for advice about how to control the spread of disease and whether the situation constitutes an outbreak. During an identified outbreak, a child or staff member will be excluded if an official in the health department or a primary care practitioner suspects that the child or staff member is contributing to the spread of the illness in the facility or lacks necessary immunization during an outbreak of a vaccine-preventable disease, or the infectious disease involved poses a special risk to that individual. Readmission for such exclusions is permitted when the health department official or primary health care professional determines that the risk is no longer present.^{CFOC3 Std. 3.6.1.4}

2. Plan for Seasonal and Pandemic Influenza (Flu)^{CFOC3 Std. 9.2.4.4}

a. **Developing a Plan for Dealing With Influenza:** A committee with representatives of staff members, parents/guardians, and a child care health consultant meets in September each year and thereafter as needed to develop/review the plan for dealing with flu.

_____

TITLE/NAME OF STAFF MEMBER

convenes the committee, collects reliable information about the seasonal flu or pandemic flu outbreak as it affects the facility, and monitors public health announcements with the help of the child care health consultant. Key information is shared with the flu committee, all staff members, and all parents/legal guardians of enrolled children. To the extent that it is feasible, communications will be in the language that all the individuals to be informed understand most easily. Committee members check with staff members and parents to be sure they receive and understand the information shared with them about flu.

b. The communication plan is as follows:

i. _____

   TITLE AND CONTACT INFORMATION

   has the legal authority to close child care programs if there is a public health emergency or pandemic.

ii. The key agencies and contact information that regulate child care and how they plan to address seasonal or pandemic influenza are

   _____

   KEY AGENCIES AND CONTACT INFORMATION.

iii. This facility maintains operations during a pandemic flu outbreak by

   _____

   MEASURES PROGRAM WILL USE FOR CONTINUITY OF BUSINESS OPERATION OF THE PROGRAM IF PROGRAM MUST CLOSE OR LIMIT ATTENDANCE.

iv. _____

   TITLE/NAME OF STAFF MEMBER

   sends reminders to families to have arrangements for backup care if the program must close in a pandemic flu outbreak.

v. Sources of subsidized meals for children in families with low income who receive meals at the child care facility if the facility must close are

   _____

   SOURCES OF SUBSIDIZED MEALS.

vi. Sources of mental health services to cope with stress during a pandemic are

   _____

   SOURCES OF MENTAL HEALTH SERVICES.

vii. Other child care programs with whom we exchange information are

   _____

   NAMES AND CONTACT INFORMATION FOR PROGRAMS WITH WHICH THIS PROGRAM SHARES INFORMATION.

viii. Keeping in touch with staff members and families during the flu outbreak or pandemic involves

_____

METHOD OF MAINTAINING COMMUNICATION.

ix. _____

TITLE/NAME OF STAFF MEMBER

sends reminders that seasonal flu vaccine; covering a sneeze or cough with a tissue, shoulder, or elbow; and practicing hand hygiene help prevent the spread of flu.

x. _____

TITLE/NAME OF STAFF MEMBER

sends reminders about contacting a health care professional as soon as a child or an adult is suspected of having the flu to see if it is possible to reduce the severity with antiviral medication.

xi. Annually,

_____

TITLE/NAME OF STAFF MEMBER

searches the following Web sites for information about flu and pandemic flu: www.cdc.gov/flu, www.flu.gov, www.aap.org/en-us/advocacy-and-policy/aap-health-initiatives/Children-and-Disasters/Pages/Preparing-Child-Care-Programs-for-Pandemic-Influenza.aspx.

c. **Infection Control Plan:** In the event of an outbreak, this facility will

i. Rigidly observe keeping children in contact only with teachers/caregivers and children in their own group.

ii. Strictly observe hand and surface hygiene measures.

iii. Use the daily health check to exclude children from attending the child care facility according to the facility exclusion policy. (See Appendix M: Instructions for Daily Health Check and Section 11.A: Admission and Exclusion.)

iv. Teach staff members and parents/guardians how to limit the spread of flu with vaccines, beginning in September and continuing until everyone has received immunizations into March or April—especially for children and adolescents 6 months to 18 years of age, teachers/caregivers, and parents/family members of children younger than 5 years. Our facility _____ that all

ENCOURAGES/REQUIRES

family members older than 6 months and all staff members receive flu vaccine as soon as it becomes available in our community unless an individual has a valid medical reason not to do so.

v. Support staff members who are ill so they can stay at home until they are well again with paid sick leave of

_____

PROVISION FOR AVAILABLE SICK LEAVE.

vi. _____
  TITLE/NAME OF STAFF MEMBER

has a plan for handling staff absences and program closings that includes substitutes for staff members who are ill, advising families how to continue their child's learning if the program is closed, meeting payroll, communicating with staff members and families, and modifications to the program if the program must be reduced or closed.

Reference

1.   American Academy of Pediatrics. *Managing Infectious Diseases in Child Care and Schools: A Quick Reference Guide.* 3rd ed. Aronson SS, Shope TR, eds. Elk Grove Village, IL: American Academy of Pediatrics; 2013

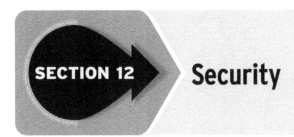

Rationale

Facilities where children are in care must guard against intrusion by individuals intending, threatening, or actually engaging in criminal or dangerous behavior. Facilities must be sure that children do not leave the building without supervision.

Required Action/Who Is Responsible/How Communicated

A. Background Screening for All Workers[CFOC3 Std. 1.2.0.2]

All staff members, employed or volunteer, regular or substitute, receive background screening that includes criminal record checks, founded reports of child abuse and neglect, references, and credential checks before they are allowed on the premises when children are present. (See Section 16.A: Background Screening for All Workers.)

B. Prevention of Access by Threatening Individuals and Sign-in, Sign-out System[CFOC3 Stds. 9.2.4.7–9.2.4.10]

1. **Entrances:** Facility entrances are observed by a staff member and maintained locked from the outside but easily opened from the inside by school-aged children or adults. An alarm is activated when a door is opened from the inside other than the monitored entrance/exit door so that no one can leave the building unnoticed.[CFOC3 Std. 5.1.4.4] The security system includes an alarm if anyone gains entrance without being recognized by

   _____

   TITLE/NAME OF STAFF MEMBER.

   _____

   TITLE(S)/NAME(S) OF STAFF MEMBER(S)

   are the only ones authorized to operate the security system and monitor entrances to the building and the doors from the reception area into child care areas.

2. **Outdoor Play Areas:** The location and layout of outdoor play areas are intended to prevent easy access by strangers or vehicles from the street. In addition, the areas are protected by fences with gates that reduce the potential for a child to exit without an adult.

3. **Access for Families:** Families are encouraged to come into the facility and go to any part where their child is in care. To gain entrance, families, staff members, and visitors

---

PROCEDURE FOR RECOGNITION OF PEOPLE WHO SHOULD BE ALLOWED TO ENTER THE RECEPTION AREA AND SUBSEQUENTLY, UNLESS THEIR BEHAVIOR INDICATES OTHERWISE, ALLOWED TO ENTER THE CHILD CARE AREA.

The staff members have a way to signal for help if anyone displays threatening behavior.

C. Sign-in/Sign-out Procedure

1. **Who Must Follow the Sign-in/Sign-out Procedure:** Without exception, everyone who enters and exits the facility must use the sign-in/sign-out procedure.

2. **Method of Documentation:** To document name, contact number, reason for being in the facility (eg, parent/legal guardian, enrolled child, visitor, vendor, consultant), and time in and out of the facility,

---

DESCRIBE METHOD USED AS A HANDWRITTEN RECORD, ELECTRONIC METHOD.

3. **Pickup of a Child**

   a. **Authorized Individuals:** Individuals authorized to take a child who is receiving care in the facility out of the facility's supervision are listed in the child's file along with that person's photograph, signature, and relationship to the child.

   b. **Identification of Authorized Individuals Before Release of a Child:** No child will be released to anyone who is not positively identified by the teacher/caregiver who is supervising the child and verified with documentation by

---

TITLE/NAME OF STAFF MEMBER

   if the person is not recognized by the teacher/caregiver.

   c. **Custody/Court Orders:** Custody issues or court orders will be copied, made known to staff members, honored, and kept on file.[CFOC3 Std. 9.2.4.8]

   d. **Extenuating Circumstances:** In an extenuating circumstance, when an authorized person cannot pick up the child, another individual may pick up a child from child care if that person is authorized to do so by the parent/guardian in authenticated communication, such as a witnessed phone conversation in which the caller provides prespecified identifying information (eg, a secret word) or written consent from the parent/legal guardian with prespecified identifying information, and confirmed by a return call to the parent/legal guardian before release of the child.[CFOC3 Std. 9.2.4.8]

   e. **Unauthorized Individual:** If an unauthorized individual arrives requesting access to the facility without the facility receiving prior communication from the child's parent/guardian, the parent/guardian should be contacted immediately, preferably privately. If the information provided by the parent/guardian does not match the information and identification of the unauthorized individual, the child will not be permitted to leave the child care facility. If it is determined that the parent/guardian is unaware of the individual's attempt to pick up the child or if the parent/guardian has not or will not authorize the individual to take the child from the child care facility, information about the individual should be documented and the individual should be asked to leave. If the individual does not leave and his or her behavior is concerning to staff members or if the child is abducted by force, the police will be contacted immediately and given a detailed description of the individual and any other obtainable information such as a license plate number.[CFOC3 Std. 9.2.4.8]

f. **Impaired or Noncustodial Parent/Legal Guardian:** If a parent/legal guardian arrives who is intoxicated or otherwise incapable of bringing the child home safely or if a noncustodial parent attempts to claim the child without consent of the custodial parent, a staff member will call the police to handle the situation. Child protective services may become involved at that point.

D. Action When No Authorized Person Arrives to Pick Up a Child[CFOC3 Std. 9.2.4.9]

1. Efforts to Contact Each Authorized Contact:

_____
TITLE/NAME OF STAFF MEMBER

will attempt to reach each authorized contact listed in the child's record. If these efforts fail, the facility will

_____
DESCRIBE WHERE THE CHILD WILL GO, WITH WHOM, AND FOR WHAT AMOUNT OF TIME BEFORE CHILD PROTECTIVE SERVICES IS NOTIFIED.

2. Repeated Failure to Meet Agreed Pickup Arrangement: A second episode of failure to pick up the child as expected will result in

_____
INDICATE DISCIPLINARY ACTION SUCH AS A FINE.

Any subsequent episodes will result in a consultation with child protective services.

E. Communications and Documentation About Attendance[CFOC3 Std. 9.2.4.10]

1. Daily Attendance Record: A daily attendance record is maintained at the entrance to the facility for all the children in the facility. This documentation identifies the arrival in the facility and departure from the facility and the person who brings and picks up the child. It is separate from daily attendance notes kept by the teachers/caregivers for the child's group for each child that lists the times of transfer of care to and from the teachers/caregivers who are supervising the child's group. (See Appendix N: Enrollment/Attendance/ Symptom Record.) The daily attendance record is kept

_____
WHERE THE DAILY ATTENDANCE RECORD IS KEPT JUST INSIDE THE FACILITY'S ENTRANCE/EXIT DOOR

and is monitored by

_____
WHO IS RESPONSIBLE FOR COMPLETING AND KEEPING TRACK OF THE COMPLETION OF THE DAILY ATTENDANCE RECORD IN THE EVENT OF A PLANNED FIELD TRIP OR EMERGENCY REMOVAL OF THE CHILD FROM THE FACILITY.

2. Notice of Planned Nonattendance: Parents/legal guardians must inform the child's teachers/caregivers by the time the child is expected to arrive if the child is not coming to the program. The child's teacher/caregiver will contact the parent/legal guardian within an hour of delayed arrival if the parent/legal guardian has not informed the program that the child will be absent. The communication can be by phone, e-mail, or text.

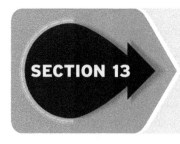

Emergencies and Disasters

Rationale

In an emergency situation, it is difficult for many people to stay calm and think clearly. Having a well-understood, practiced, and performed emergency plan guides good decision-making under stress. Unannounced mock drills of different types of emergencies help build competence and confidence and identify parts of the plan and procedures that need to be revised.

Required Action/Who Is Responsible/How Communicated

A. Urgent Medical or Oral Health Care

1. First Aid Kits

    a. Location of First Aid Kits: A fully stocked first aid kit is located in every room or other location where children are in care. The kits are in a closed container, cabinet, or drawer that is labeled, known, and always accessible to all staff but not to children.^{CFOC3 Std. 5.6.0.1}

    b. Restocking of First Aid Kits:

TITLE/NAME OF STAFF MEMBER

    restocks first aid kits after each use, checks the contents monthly for missing or expired items, and completes a log indicating the date and actions taken as a result of the first aid kit check using the inventory of items that should be in the kit. (See Appendix BB: First Aid Kit Inventory.)

    c. Location of Emergency Medications: If any child in the group requires emergency medication (eg, EpiPen, metered-dose inhaler for asthma, antihistamine for allergic reaction), the medication is kept in the first aid kit where the child is in care (if the kit can be kept handy but locked to be sure it is inaccessible to children) or carried in a fanny pack by the teacher/caregiver who is supervising the child.

    d. First Aid Kits for Trips: Teachers/caregivers take an appropriately supplied first aid kit on trips (walking or vehicular) to and from the facility and playground.

2. First Aid and CPR Training for Staff ^{CFOC3 Stds. 1.4.3}

    a. Staff Members Must Document Satisfactory Completion of First Aid and CPR Training:

TITLE/NAME OF STAFF MEMBER

    ensures that all staff members involved in providing direct care have documentation of satisfactory completion of pediatric first aid and cardiopulmonary resuscitation (CPR) training that is renewed as required by the organization providing the training. Cardiopulmonary resuscitation training must include demonstration, practice, and return demonstration to ensure that the technique can be properly performed in an emergency. Personnel files of the facility hold the documentation of successful completion of pediatric first aid and CPR training.

b. **Topics Covered in First Aid/CPR Training:** Topics included in first aid and CPR training include an overview of emergency medical services (EMS); how to access EMS; the poison center; ensuring safety at the scene; management of body substances; management of blocked airway and rescue breathing; care of abrasions, lacerations, bleeding including nosebleeds, burns, fainting, poisoning (swallowed, skin contact, eye contact, inhaled), puncture wounds including splinters, bites (insects, animal, human), shock, seizures, musculoskeletal injuries (sprains, fractures), oral injuries, head injuries, allergic reactions including when and how to use injected epinephrine, asthma including when and how to use inhalers, eye injuries, electric shock, drowning, heat-related illnesses, and cold-related injuries (frost nip, frostbite); moving and positioning people who are injured or ill; illness-related emergencies (eg, stiff neck, inexplicable confusion, sudden onset of blood red or purple rash, severe pain, elevated body temperature accompanied by looking very ill); Standard Precautions; following the plan for emergency care of any child in the group who has a special need; and addressing the needs of the other children in the group while managing an emergency.

3. **Management of Injuries or Illnesses That Require Medical or Oral Health Professional Care**

a. **Calling 911:** The teacher/caregiver who is supervising the child or with the adult who is injured or ill will call 911 or ask

_____

TITLE/NAME OF STAFF MEMBER

to immediately call 911.

b. **Contacting Parents/Legal Guardians:**

_____

TITLE/NAME OF STAFF MEMBER

will contact the parent/legal guardian of a child who is ill or injured. If the parent/legal guardian cannot be reached or the person who is ill or injured is an adult, an emergency contact person listed in the facility files will be contacted.

c. **Closest Emergency Medical Facility:** The closest emergency medical facility to the program for children is

_____

NAME OF FACILITY

and for adults is

_____

NAME OF FACILITY.

Prior to a specific medical emergency,

_____

TITLE/NAME OF STAFF MEMBER

contacts emergency facilities to find out what procedures the emergency facility follows when EMS brings a child who is not accompanied by a parent/legal guardian or an adult who may not be able to communicate.

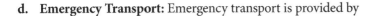

    d. **Emergency Transport:** Emergency transport is provided by

_____

IDENTIFY EMS SERVICE WITH PHONE NUMBER.

    e. **Staff Member Escort to Emergency Care:** A staff member accompanies and remains with the child or adult who is ill or injured until the parent/legal guardian or other responsible party assumes responsibility.

_____

TITLE/NAME OF STAFF MEMBER

    makes sure that child:staff ratios are maintained at all times for the children remaining in the facility.

    f. **Incident Reports:** The staff member who provided first aid completes an incident report form as soon after the incident as possible. (See Appendix CC: Incident Report Form.)

_____

TITLE/NAME OF STAFF MEMBER

    makes sure that the form is signed by the parent/legal guardian or the injured adult and distributes copies to 1) the parent/legal guardian or adult who is ill or injured, 2) the child's or teacher's/caregiver's record at the facility, and 3) the facility's incident log or file.

    g. **Oral Health Emergencies:** After or while a staff member provides first aid for an oral injury,

_____

TITLE/NAME OF STAFF MEMBER

    contacts

_____

ORAL HEALTH PROFESSIONAL/PRACTICE NAME

    the licensed oral health professional who has agreed to accept emergency dental referrals of children from this facility and give advice on a dental emergency. If the parent/legal guardian has an oral health professional who provides emergency advice and care, the staff member will use this contact first. If emergency dental care is required, a staff member accompanies the child and remains with the child until the parent/legal guardian assumes responsibility for the child.

B. Emergency/Urgent Contact and Health Information

1. Access to Emergency Contact and Health Information:

_____

TITLE/NAME OF STAFF MEMBER

ensures that emergency contact and health care information for each child and volunteer or employed staff member is readily available when children or adults are engaged in activities on-site or off-site. A copy of this information will be available and given to EMS in a medical emergency.*CFOC3 Std. 9.4.2.2*

2. **Updating and Verifying Emergency Contact and Health Information:** Emergency contact and health information is updated and verified by calling the numbers quarterly. For children, this information includes work addresses and emergency phone numbers or other means of rapid contact for parents/legal guardians and 2 alternate emergency contacts, contact information for the child's primary health care professional, and health information relevant to care in an emergency. For adults, this information includes a next of kin and an alternate emergency contact, the primary health care professional, and health information relevant to care in an emergency.

C. Emergency Repairs

_____

TITLE/NAME OF STAFF MEMBER

maintains contact information for contractors who provide specific types of building repairs for this facility. These are kept in

_____

LOCATION.

_____

TITLE/NAME OF STAFF MEMBER

calls appropriate contractors for problems with electricity, heating, plumbing, snow removal, trash removal, and general maintenance.

D. Serious Illness, Hospitalization, and Death

1. **Attention to Child Witnesses:** If a child or an adult has an event related to a serious physical or mental illness or injury or dies while in the facility, the teacher/caregiver responsible for anyone who observed or was in the same room where the death/injury occurred removes the children to another room while giving minimal but reassuring comments. Other staff members tend to the situation.

2. **Notification of EMS and Next of Kin:**

_____

TITLE(S)/NAME(S) OF STAFF MEMBER(S)

will immediately call EMS and notify the child's parents/legal guardians or adult's emergency contact person to come where professionals skilled in informing about such events are available.

_____

TITLE(S)/NAME(S) OF STAFF MEMBER(S)

will communicate with staff, families, children, and the community about the event.

3. Controlling the Scene, Subsequent Communications, and Support:

_____
TITLE(S)/NAME(S) OF STAFF MEMBER(S)

make sure nothing is done to disturb a death scene or show it to or talk about it with others. Thereafter, depending on the nature of the death (eg, sudden infant death syndrome, medical event, injury),

_____
TITLE(S)/NAME(S) OF STAFF MEMBER(S)

make available supportive resources for everyone who knows about the event. Specific information about the event is only released to those whom the authorities and family agree should have these details.[CFOC3 Std. 3.6.4.5] Each action taken is documented in the facility records.

4. Notification of Agencies and Authorities:

_____
TITLE/NAME OF STAFF MEMBER

will immediately notify

_____
NAME OF ANY REQUIRED AGENCIES SUCH AS THE POLICE, HEALTH DEPARTMENT, OR STATE REGULATING AGENCY

of a serious injury/illness that requires emergency department care/hospitalization or results in the death of a child or staff member that occurs during the child care day or related to any child care activity.

_____
TITLE/NAME OF STAFF MEMBER

ensure that full documentation of all events and actions taken is prepared and kept in the facility files.[CFOC3 Std. 9.4.1.10]

E. Lost or Missing Children

1. Counting and Identifying Location of Each Child: To prevent lost or missing children, staff count children with a face-and-head count at least every 15 minutes.

_____
TITLE/NAME OF STAFF MEMBER

is responsible for performing a sweep of the child care facility when everyone has left the building and any vehicle in which children are leaving to be sure that no child is overlooked.

2. Prevention and Recovery of Missing Children:

_____
TITLE/NAME OF STAFF MEMBER

will implement specific systems for prevention and speedy recovery of missing children. For example, on field trips, every child and staff member might wear uniform, brightly colored T-shirts with an attached pocket that holds the child's identification and program's contact information. This information will not be easily viewed by a stranger who might use the child's name to lure the child from the group. With consent from the parent/legal guardian, staff will carry a picture of each child when off-site to aid others to help locate a child. Staff members will give instructions to older children about what to do if they separate from the group.

3. Procedure for Unrecovered Missing or Lost Children: If it is determined that a child is missing or lost,

_____
TITLE/NAME OF STAFF MEMBER

immediately notify the local police or sheriff, program director, parents/legal guardians, and other authorities as required by state regulation. If on a field trip, the staff will notify the facility management to assist in the search for the child.[CFOC3 Std. 9.2.4.1]

F. Emergency and Evacuation Plan, Drills, and Closings

1. Emergency Preparedness Planning: This facility has planned for emergencies using the approach outlined in the Head Start Emergency Preparedness Manual found at http://eclkc.ohs.acf.hhs.gov/hslc/standards/IMs/2009/resour_ime_009_121409.html or in the free, on-demand distance education lessons available from Penn State University Better Kid Care at www.betterkidcare.psu.edu/page14.html. Annually, staff members review the plan, suggest any changes that need to be made, and affix their signatures to the current plan. Parents/legal guardians are encouraged to review and contribute to updating the plan also.

2. Risk Analysis Results: Our facility's risk analysis revealed the following anticipatable hazards/disasters for which we have planned:

_____
APPLICABLE RISKS FROM THE FOLLOWING LIST OF EMERGENCIES/DISASTERS: ACUTE/URGENT MEDICAL CARE AND EVACUATION OF CHILDREN AND ADULTS WHO ARE INJURED ILL (EG, SEVERE BLEEDING, UNRESPONSIVENESS, POISONING, CIRCULATORY FAILURE OR HEART ATTACK, SEIZURES, HEAD INJURIES, SEVERE ALLERGIC REACTIONS, ASTHMA, DEHYDRATION, HEAT ILLNESS), INCLUDING READINESS TO PROVIDE FIRST AID AND CPR); BOMB THREATS; EARTHQUAKE; ELECTRICAL POWER OUTAGES; EXTREME HEAT OR COLD; FAILED HEATING/COOLING SYSTEMS; FIRE; FLOOD; HURRICANE; LANDSLIDE/MUDSLIDE; PLUMBING OR SEWAGE PROBLEMS; ROAD CLOSINGS; SNOWSTORMS/BLIZZARDS; THREATENING PERSONS/CRIMINAL OR TERRORIST EVENT; TORNADO; TOXIC CHEMICALS; VOLCANO; WATER LEAKS; WILDFIRE.

3. Evacuation and Lockdown Plans: Evacuation and lockdown plans address shelter in place and evacuation to a location near the facility and to a safe place away from danger in the community or area surrounding the facility. These plans are kept in

_____
LOCATION

and reviewed with staff members annually by

_____
TITLE/NAME OF STAFF MEMBER.

4. Review of Emergency Plans:

_____

TITLE/NAME OF STAFF MEMBER

annually reviews emergency plans with

_____

RESOURCES FOR EMERGENCY PLANNING EXPERTISE INVOLVED

to update our decision trees, action checklists for shelter in place, evacuation, relocation, and long-term recovery plans for each type of hazard/disaster that might affect our facility. If our facility is involved in a disaster,

_____

TITLE/NAME OF STAFF MEMBER

will use the Child Care Initial Rapid Damage Assessment tool and apply the previously established plans as appropriate. (See Appendix DD: Child Care Initial Rapid Damage Assessment.)

5. Location and Content of Emergency Supplies: Emergency supplies are kept

_____

WHERE THE SUPPLIES ARE KEPT

and are checked for needed replacements by

_____

TITLE/NAME OF STAFF MEMBER

every 6 months or sooner if the supplies may have been used. The supplies are checked to be sure they are not outdated. Our facility _____ in an area where natural disasters occur that necessitates keeping
IS/IS NOT

at least a 72-hour supply of food and water for each child and staff member.$^{CFOC3 Std. 4.9.0.8}$

6. Emergency Contact and Health Information: Parent/legal guardian contact information and necessary information to accompany a child to an emergency medical facility when the parent/legal guardian is not available to provide information and consent for care is kept

_____

LOCATIONS.

Our facility has contacted the local EMS and hospitals that are the likely sources of emergency medical care to determine the items and format of this information that they would use. We have determined that their policy related to limitations on their acceptance of pre-incident authorizations of consent for care if a parent/legal guardian cannot be reached is

_____

CURRENT POLICY OF EMS AND HOSPITALS TO WHICH CHILDREN/ADULTS WHO ARE INJURED OR SERIOUSLY ILL WOULD BE TAKEN.

7. **Notification of Families About an Emergency:** Families are notified about an emergency by

_____

METHOD AND RESPONSIBLE STAFF MEMBER(S) WHO WILL NOTIFY FAMILIES.

Information about the evacuation will be given to

_____

LOCAL EMERGENCY MEDIA SOURCE CALL NUMBERS/STATION NAME

while individual notification of families is underway so families can know as soon as possible what measures are being taken.

8. **Evacuation Procedure**

   a. **Child:Staff Ratios During Emergency Evacuation:** Child:staff ratios in an emergency evacuation will be maintained.

   b. **Evacuation of Children With Special Needs:** Children with special needs will be accommodated according to their special care plans.[CFOC3 Std. 5.1.4.2]

   c. **Nonambulatory Children:** Children who cannot walk out of the building on their own will be evacuated as planned in consultation with a fire safety professional.

      i. **Method Used for Infants and Toddlers:**

      _____

      DESCRIBE METHOD (EG, EVACUATION CRIB, HUMAN CHAIN WITH HAND ON THE SHOULDER IN FRONT).

      ii. **Method Used for Children With Disabilities:**

      _____

      DESCRIBE METHOD (EG, WHEELCHAIR, WALKING WITH CHILDREN BETWEEN STAFF, HOLDING ONTO A ROPE).

   d. **Counting Children:** Staff count the children with face-to-name recognition in each group being evacuated and count the children again when they reach the evacuation destination.

   e. **Instructions to Children:** Staff give children clear, simple instructions about exiting the facility. Children are to stop their activities immediately at the sound of the alarm and proceed to the exit door.

   f **Attendance Lists:**

   _____

   TITLE/NAME OF STAFF MEMBER

   carries attendance and emergency contact information from the facility and compares attendance to the attendance sheet to be sure no children or staff members have been left behind when they gather at[CFOC3 Std. 9.2.4.6]

   _____

   LOCATION WHERE EVACUEES WILL GATHER.

g. **Sweep of All Areas:** To ensure complete evacuation has occurred, the last person to leave each part of the facility conducts a final, thorough sweep of all areas accessible to children (whether or not children are allowed in those areas). The facility posts a list in each area to be checked as part of the sweep in each part of the facility. The last person to leave will use the list of accessible areas to check each area and then take the list to

_____

LOCATION WHERE EVACUEES WILL GATHER.

Each person who conducted a sweep signs the list of areas checked and gives the list to

_____

TITLE/NAME OF STAFF MEMBER.

If a child who should have been evacuated with the group is located as a result of a final sweep during an evacuation drill, the director will investigate the circumstances that led to the failure to evacuate that child and plan how to avoid such problems in the future.

h. **Staff Assignments:**

_____

TITLE/NAME OF STAFF MEMBER

checks quarterly that each staff member knows a specific assignment in an emergency.

i. **Temporary Shelter:** If reentry into the building is not possible, children will be evacuated to

_____

NAME AND LOCATION OF NEARBY TEMPORARY SHELTER TO BE USED IN AN EMERGENCY OR LOCATION OF SHELTER A SAFE DISTANCE FROM A DISASTER AREA.

(See appendixes EE: Sample Letter of Agreement With Emergency Evacuation Site and FF: Sample Letter to Parents About Evacuation Arrangements.) Staff will remain calm and speak to the children in a reassuring manner. The temporary shelter is stocked, or program staff members bring an emergency supplies list to the temporary shelter with supplies and materials for

_____

NUMBER OF HOURS OR DAYS

the maximum time that this program believes might be necessary for the program to take care of children until parents/legal guardians or designated persons can take children home.

j. **Locations Where Evacuation Procedures Are Posted:** Evacuation procedures are posted in the facility at

_____

LOCATIONS.

9. Emergency Drills*CFOC3* Std. 9.2.4.5

   a. **Evacuation Drills:** Evacuation drills for fire are held monthly. For other emergencies that may require evacuation, drills are held

   ---

   AS APPROPRIATE TO THE NATURALLY OCCURRING DISASTERS IN THE FACILITY'S LOCATION: MONTHLY IN TORNADO SEASON, BEFORE THE FLOOD SEASON, EVERY 6 MONTHS FOR EARTHQUAKES, ANNUALLY FOR HURRICANES.

   At least one drill includes evacuation to a temporary shelter away from the facility. Other drills include what needs to be done for other hazardous/risk situations identified in the risk analysis, including a drill to practice how to deal with a threatening individual.

   b. **Drills for Emergency Events That May Require Shelter in Place:** Drills are held annually for a threatening person outside or inside the facility, a stray animal or one that appears sick, a toxic chemical spill, and a nuclear event. At least one drill each year involves shelter in place.

   c. **Timing and Documentation of Drills:** Timing of the drills will be varied to include early morning, mealtimes, and nap times.

   TITLE/NAME OF STAFF MEMBER

   complete the Evacuation Drill Log at the end of each drill. (See Appendix GG: Evacuation Drill Log.)

   d. **Preparation of Children for Drills:** Children will be appropriately prepared for and reassured during drills. If shoes are removed for nap time, they are kept where they can be easily carried out and put on the children when they are safely out of the building.

   e. **Observation of Drills by an Emergency Preparedness Professional:** At least one drill per year will be observed by a representative of the fire department or equivalent emergency or community disaster planning professional. Annually,

   ---

   TITLE/NAME OF STAFF MEMBER

   will ask the community disaster planning professional to review the Evacuation Drill Log and suggest any possible improvements in the facility's procedure.*CFOC3* Std. 9.4.1.16

10. Emergency Training for New Staff:

   TITLE/NAME OF STAFF MEMBER

   provides all new staff preservice training about emergency plans. Emergency plans are shared with new staff by or on the first day of employment.*CFOC3* Std. 1.4.1.1

G. Media Inquiries

   • All media inquiries are referred to

   TITLE/NAME OF STAFF MEMBER.

   • Media representatives are not allowed access to the facility during a crisis situation.
   • Media access will be prearranged at times when staff members and families have been informed and when such visits will cause the least amount of disruption to the program.

Child Abuse and Neglect (Child Maltreatment)^{CFOC3} Std. 3.4.4

Rationale

All adults who work in child care must be aware of the common physical and emotional signs and symptoms of child abuse and neglect, also called child maltreatment. State law mandates reporting suspected child maltreatment to child protective services or the police. While laws vary from state to state, in all states, failing to report is a crime that may result in legal penalties. State laws protect well-intended reporters of suspected child maltreatment from adverse consequences of making reports, even if the suspected child abuse is not confirmed by the investigation triggered by the report. Commonly, reporting suspected maltreatment initiates support for families under stress whether or not the investigation determines that their children are abused or neglected.

Required Action/Who Is Responsible/How Communicated

A. Preventing Overwhelming Situations

1. **Relief for Stressed Staff Members:** Teachers/caregivers and all others who are involved with children are expected to ask for relief from duty by

   _____

   METHOD TO REQUEST RELIEF

   when feeling overwhelmed or stressed to avoid situations in which a child might be abused. Teachers/caregivers have stress-relief breaks of no less than 15 minutes every 4 hours and at least a 30-minute break for or after a meal.

2. **Care for Stressed Children:** No child is shaken, hit, or handled in a way that causes emotional or physical pain. Adults comfort and remove from stressful situations children who are crying, fussing, acting distressed, or hurting others. (See also Section 3.B: Permissible Methods for Teaching, Behavior Management, and Discipline.)

B. Layout and Staffing to Reduce the Risk of Child Abuse or Neglect

1. **Visibility of All Activities:** The layout of this facility is intended to provide a high level of visibility outside and inside, including diapering and toileting areas used by children. All areas can be viewed by at least one other adult in addition to an individual teacher/caregiver at all times when children are in care. The facility uses windows into rooms from hallways and mirrors to see into otherwise difficult-to-view areas.

2. **Two Adults Per Group:** Two adults are present in each area to the extent such staffing is possible.

3. **Limiting Privacy:** Unannounced visits by other staff members are frequent when a teacher/caregiver is alone, and set up of furnishings limit isolation and privacy where children might be undressed or nude to reduce the risk of child abuse or neglect or unwarranted suspicion of child abuse or neglect.

C. Mandated Reporters of Child Abuse or Neglect

1. **Who Is a Mandated Reporter:** Teachers/caregivers and most others who are in any way involved in a program that cares for children are mandated reporters of suspected child abuse and neglect, no matter where the child maltreatment occurred.

2. **Where to Report Suspected Abuse or Neglect:** Anyone in the facility who thinks child abuse or neglect has occurred must report this suspicion to the child abuse reporting hotline. The phone number for the child abuse hot line is

   _____

   HOTLINE NUMBER.

   The person making the report will follow the guidance of the child protective services agency concerning notification of the parent/legal guardian of the child involved in the report and any further reporting required by law.

3. **Protection of the Mandated Reporter:** No disciplinary or retaliatory action is taken against anyone who makes a report of suspected child abuse or neglect unless a false report was knowingly made.

4. **Staff Members Suspected of Child Maltreatment:** Staff members who are alleged to be perpetrators of child maltreatment may be suspended or given leave _____ pending completion of an
   WITH/WITHOUT PAY

   investigation or may be removed from contact with children and given a job that does not require interaction with children.

   _____

   TITLE/NAME OF STAFF MEMBER

   informs parents/legal guardians of children who may have been victims of maltreatment in the facility and parents/legal guardians of other children in the program that an unconfirmed concern about child maltreatment is being investigated. This informing will not mention the names of the parties involved. As part of the informing, the staff member making the contact invites parents/guardians to share any concerns they have had about the care of their own children. No accusation or affirmation of guilt is made until the investigation is complete. Any teacher/caregiver found guilty of child maltreatment will be dismissed.

5. **Documentation of Observations:** It is not necessary to have evidence to support reporting a suspicion of child abuse or neglect. However, it is best to document observations, such as bruises or what the child says in play about being abused, in the facility's records. Forms provided by the state/county children and youth services to document observations and information for making a child abuse or neglect report are available. The forms are kept

   _____

   LOCATION OF FORMS.

   _____

   TITLE/NAME OF STAFF MEMBER

   can help fill out the forms and make a report if asked to do so.

D. Training and Supportive Resources About Child Abuse and Neglect

1. **Staff Member Participation in Training About Child Abuse and Neglect:** Everyone in the facility must participate in initial and ongoing training to prevent, recognize, and report signs of child abuse and neglect. (See Appendix HH: What Is Child Abuse and Neglect? Recognizing the Signs and Symptoms.)

2. **Arrangements for Child Abuse and Neglect Training:**

   _____
   TITLE/NAME OF STAFF MEMBER

   arranges or identifies opportunities to receive the required training.

3. **Source of Specialized Resources and Training to Care for Children Who Have Experienced Child Abuse or Neglect:** Specialized resources and training for teachers/caregivers in management of children who have been abused or neglected are available from

   _____
   LOCAL CHILD PROTECTIVE SERVICES AGENCY NAME AND CONTACT INFORMATION OR PEDIATRIC MENTAL HEALTH OR OTHER ALTERNATIVE RESOURCE.

E. Informing Parents/Legal Guardians About Mandated Reporting

_____
TITLE/NAME OF STAFF MEMBER

is responsible for making sure each parent/legal guardian is informed at the time of a child's admission to the facility about the mandated reporting responsibility.

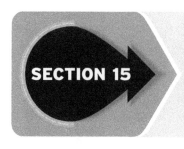

Smoking, Prohibited Substances, and Weapons

Rationale

Children must be protected from exposure to toxic substances, illegal drugs, medications not intended for the user, and weapons. Each of these poses a significant risk of injury to children.

Secondhand smoke is in the air around a smoker. Toxic products in secondhand smoke enter the airways of others who are in the same space as a smoker. Secondhand smoke exposure is harmful. In addition, thirdhand smoke exposure occurs because smoke products cling to the hair, clothing, and surfaces wherever someone has smoked, even if the smoker is not smoking when others are in the same space as the smoker. These smoke products also contain harmful toxic substances. Children can get these substances on their hands when they play on the floor or touch other surfaces. These toxins can irritate sensitive airways and trigger asthma and allergies.

Other substances such as alcohol and illegal and legal drugs that impair clear thinking and responsible behavior can lead to poor-quality care for children.

Children are curious and likely to investigate any weapon they find, no matter how much they are cautioned against doing so. Children have limited ability to understand the risks and proper use of weapons and the real-life consequences of behaviors involving weapons. The result can be severe injury and death involving themselves or others.

Required Action/Who Is Responsible/How Communicated

A. Prohibited Substances

1. **Adherence to Policies Related to Prohibited Substances:** Smoking of any kind or wearing of clothing with smoke residues; use of tobacco products, alcohol, and illegal drugs; and unauthorized use of potentially toxic substances are all prohibited in this facility, on facility grounds, in any vehicles that transport children, or whenever a staff member is supervising children in off-site play areas and on field trips away from the facility.[CFOC3 Stds. 3.4.1.1, 9.2.3.15] Violators of this policy will be disciplined by

_____

SPECIFY TITLE/NAME OF STAFF MEMBER WHO DECIDES AND ENFORCES DISCIPLINARY MEASURES.

   a. **People Who Smoke Off Premises:** Because toxins from tobacco smoke are in the fabrics worn and used in the environment of smokers, any employee or volunteer who smokes is required to change into clean clothing on arrival at the facility. (For family child care homes, there is no smoking by anyone at any time in the facility.)

   b. **Exclusion of Workers Who Are Impaired:** Workers in this facility are expected to refrain from the use of alcohol or any drugs that may impair their ability to perform their job for as long as is required not to affect their behavior or abilities at work. Teachers/caregivers, other staff members, or other adults who are inebriated, intoxicated, or otherwise under the influence of mind-altering or other substances that can result in harm to others will be required to leave the premises immediately.

2. Informing Adults About Prohibited Substances:

TITLE/NAME OF STAFF MEMBER

is responsible for providing information available to all adults who work in or visit the facility during the hours of operation or at other times about prohibited substances (eg, maintenance contractors, individuals who share use of the facility at times when the program is not operating).

TITLE/NAME OF STAFF MEMBER

provides information about available drug, alcohol, and tobacco cessation support programs and any available employee assistance programs to anyone who is involved in any way with the program. This includes posting signs as reminders about prohibited substances and making handouts or other educational materials available about cessation support programs.

B. Weapons

1. **Specific Types of Prohibited Items:** No weapons of any type are permitted on the facility premises or anywhere being used for activities that are part of the facility's program. Prohibited items include firearms, pellet guns, BB guns, darts, bows and arrows, cap pistols, stun guns, paintball guns, ammunition, explosive devices, knives or any type of supplies intended for use as weapons, and any objects manufactured as toy versions of these weapons.[CFOC3 Std. 5.5.0.8]

2. **Response to Any Attempt to Bring a Weapon Into the Facility:** Anyone who attempts to enter or gains entry to the facility and has a prohibited item will leave the facility premises immediately.

TITLE/NAME OF STAFF MEMBER

calls the police without delay if anyone attempts to violate this policy.

Human Resources/Personnel Policies^{CFOC3 Std. 9.3.0.1}

Rationale

Children must be protected from exposure to individuals who lack the necessary credentials and experience or have a history of abuse or neglect that disqualifies them from being where children are in care. Diligent background screening protects everyone involved with the child care program from difficult and potentially criminal activity within the workforce of the facility. Workers in child care facilities should be expected to comply with policies and receive respect, recognition, and compensation at a level commensurate with the high societal value of their work.

Required Action/Who Is Responsible/How Communicated

A. Background Screening

1. **Enforcing Background Screening:**

   _____
   TITLE/NAME OF STAFF MEMBER

   is responsible for informing and ensuring that before anyone works in this facility in any role related to any activity where children are present that background screening is done.^{CFOC3 Std. 1.2.0.2}

2. **Background Screening Includes Verification of Each Individual's Information:**
   a. **Items to Be Provided by the Individual and Then Verified:**
      i. Name, address, and any other contact information
      ii. Social security number
      iii. Education
      iv. Employment history
      v. References from previous employers or supervisors who are unrelated to the candidate
   b. **Items to Be Verified by Contacting Government Agencies:**
      i. Social security trace to identify past addresses and aliases used
      ii. Driving history from Department of Motor Vehicles records
      iii. Search of state and national criminal history records accessed as advised by law enforcement authorities using court records and fingerprints
      iv. Search of records of child abuse or neglect and sex offender registries

B. Staff Health Assessment

All staff members (volunteer and paid) who have any contact with children or with anything with which children come into contact must have an initial, job-related health assessment performed within the 4-month period that begins 3 months before the employment date and ends 1 month after the employment date. (See Appendix W: Child Care Staff Health Assessment.) Subsequent health assessments are required as outlined in Section 10.A.2: Adult Health Assessment.

C. Benefits *CFOC3 Stds. 1.4.6.1, 1.4.6.2, 1.8.1.1*

1. Medical Insurance:

_____

COVERAGE ARRANGEMENTS.

2. Vacation and Holidays:

_____

AMOUNT OF ANNUAL LEAVE AND DEFINE HOLIDAYS, HOW TO APPLY FOR AND RECEIVE AUTHORIZED LEAVE.

3. Sick Leave:

_____

DAYS/YEAR OF SICK LEAVE, HOW TO NOTIFY ABOUT THE NEED AND RECEIVE AUTHORIZATION TO USE THIS LEAVE.

4. Retirement Benefits:

_____

PLAN.

5. Personal and Family Medical Leave:

_____

DAYS/YEAR OF LEAVE, HOW TO MAKE REQUESTS AND RECEIVE AUTHORIZATION FOR THIS LEAVE.

6. Substitutes for Allowed Absences:

_____

LIST CIRCUMSTANCES (EG, TRAINING, AUTHORIZED LEAVE REQUESTS) FOR WHICH SUBSTITUTES ARE PROVIDED.

7. Other Benefits:

_____

WORKERS' COMPENSATION, PARENTAL LEAVE, REDUCED CHILD CARE FEES, LIFE INSURANCE, EDUCATION, AND ANY OTHER BENEFITS FOR WHICH EMPLOYEES ARE ELIGIBLE.

D. Breaks and Stress Management^{CFOC3 Std. 1.7.0.5}

1. **Staff Entitlement to Breaks:** All staff members are entitled to breaks of

_____

AMOUNT OF BREAK TIME (AT LEAST 15 MINUTES)

for each (no more than 4 hours)

_____

NUMBER OF CONSECUTIVE HOURS WORKED BEFORE TAKING A ROUTINE BREAK (NO MORE THAN 4 HOURS)

and

_____

ANY OTHER TYPE OF BREAK.

2. **Scheduling of Breaks:**

_____

TITLE/NAME OF STAFF MEMBER

schedules all breaks.

3. **Maintenance of Child:Staff Ratios:** Breaks may be taken only if child:staff ratios for supervision of children can be maintained during the break period. If limitation of breaks is affected by insufficient staffing,

_____

TITLE/NAME OF STAFF SUPERVISOR

will be asked to solve the problem when it occurs.

4. **Stress-reduction Measures:** The administration of this facility implements the following stress-reduction measures for those who work in this program to the maximum feasible extent to ensure continuity of care and minimize job turnover rates^{CFOC3 Std. 1.7.0.5}:
   - Clear, explicit job descriptions
   - Fair compensation
   - Job security
   - Continuing education relevant to an individual's job description, including stress management
   - Regularly scheduled breaks
   - Paid time off for vacation and sick leave
   - Comfortable adult furniture in child care areas and in a staff lounge that is separate from child care areas
   - Liability insurance
   - Use of sound-absorbing materials to reduce noise-related stress
   - Regular performance reviews with constructive feedback
   - Back-up staff to maintain full complement of staff in all areas of the program

E. Professional Development/Training

1. **Compensation for Time Spent on Professional Development:** Professional development is required for all staff members (paid and volunteer) to maintain and improve their competence. Paid staff members may use paid time for professional development or receive compensation for the hours required in addition to staff members' usual schedule. Volunteers will receive recognition for their professional development efforts.[CFOC3 Std. 1.4.6.1]

2. **Preservice Training:** All new staff members (paid and volunteer, including substitutes) must receive 30 hours of orientation prior to being allowed to independently assume their job responsibilities.[CFOC3 Stds. 1.4.1] The orientation includes

   a. Goals and philosophy of the program

   b. Regulatory/accreditation/quality improvement recognition requirements

   c. Health, safety, and psychosocial issues related to child development and prevention of child abuse

   d. Operational routines in the facility including emergency procedures

   e. Reading and Review of Site-specific and Role-specific Policies:

      i. Feedback to a supervisor to test understanding of policies

      ii. Signing a document that indicates the new staff member understands and agrees to follow the written policies and procedures of the facility that are relevant to the staff member's role

   f. Names, ages, and developmental and special needs of children for whose care the staff person is involved in any way

3. **First Aid/CPR/Water Safety Training**

   a. **Documentation of Satisfactory Completion of First Aid/CPR Training:** All staff members who provide direct care of children must have current documentation of satisfactory completion of training in pediatric first aid and pediatric cardiopulmonary resuscitation (CPR) skills. Pediatric CPR skills are the same as the currently recommended approach to management of a blocked airway, the most likely life-threatening emergency event that requires CPR for a child. Pediatric CPR skills must be taught by demonstration, practice, and return demonstration to be sure that the staff member can perform the necessary actions in an emergency. In addition, the first aid training course must address all of the conditions listed in CFOC3 Standard 1.4.3.2.[CFOC3 Stds. 1.4.3.1, 1.4.3.2] (See corresponding Section 13.A.2: First Aid and CPR Training for Staff.)

   b. **Water Safety Training Requirement:** At all times when children with special needs are in care and whenever children are swimming or wading, at least one staff member must be available who is currently certified to have successfully completed training in basic water safety, proper use of swimming pool rescue equipment, and infant/child CPR.[CFOC3 Std. 1.4.3.3]

4. **Ongoing Professional Development**

   a. **Minimum Training Requirements:** Minimum training requirements for staff involved in independent direct care of children include at least 30 hours in the first year of work (16 of those 30 hours in early brain and child development and 14 hours in child health, safety, and staff health). Each year after the first year, staff are required to have at least 24 hours of continuing education based on individual needs to expand competence (16 hours in early brain and child development and 8 hours in child health, safety, and staff health).

   b. **Training Related to Performance Review:** Annually, all staff members (paid and volunteers) participate in professional development activities that enhance the quality of their performance based on their performance review.

c. **Specialized Professional Development**

i. Staff members will not take responsibility for any aspect of care for which they have not been oriented to the required knowledge and taught the necessary skills. Any staff member who is expected to care for a child with special needs reviews that child's special care plan and receives training from a licensed health care professional to perform any medical procedures or administer medication that the child requires.*CFOC3 Std. 3.5.0.2*

ii. Staff members who care for infants must receive professional development to ensure they understand and use safe sleep practices to prevent sleep-related deaths.*CFOC3 Std. 3.1.4.1*

iii. Staff members who handle food must have specialized training in safe and healthful food preparation and service.*CFOC3 Std. 1.4.5.1* This training is provided for the food handlers in this facility by

_____

AGENCY OR SOURCE OF FOOD SERVICE TRAINING.

iv. All staff members receive annual instruction related to prevention and response to suspected child abuse and neglect (child maltreatment). These educational activities include prevention and recognition of child maltreatment including physical, sexual, psychological, or emotional maltreatment; the risk of shaking infants and toddlers; and exposure of children to violence committed on others. In addition, staff members learn how to promote protective factors to prevent child maltreatment, identify signs of stress in families and teachers/caregivers, and link those who exhibit signs of stress with resources. Also, all staff members annually review with their supervisors how to carry out their legal responsibility to be a mandated reporter of suspected child abuse or neglect. (See Section 14: Child Abuse and Neglect [Child Maltreatment].)*CFOC3 Std. 1.4.5.2*

v. All staff are advised about occupational risks related to their role and how to protect themselves from these risks.*CFOC3 Std. 1.4.5.3*

vi. All staff receive education about how to adopt responsive and respectful approaches to cultural and ethnic diversity for all coworkers, families, and communities involved with the facility.*CFOC3 Std. 1.4.5.4*

F. Performance Evaluation

1. **Evaluation Procedure:** Staff members (paid and volunteer) evaluate and improve their own performance based on ongoing reflection and feedback from supervisors, peers, and families they are serving. Each person uses an annual summary of the results of these approaches to evaluation to plan her/his professional development with an immediate supervisor. This evaluation includes a review of compliance with policies and procedures of the program, level of competence in carrying out tasks identified in that person's job description, and a review of written, reflective self-evaluation.*CFOC3 Std. 1.8.2.2*

2. **Needs Assessment for Professional Development:** Supervisors conduct a needs assessment to identify areas in which supervised staff members would benefit from professional development. The needs assessment is the basis for a professional development plan for the individual and, where needs are broad-based, for multiple staff members. Supervisors measure the effectiveness of professional development by improved performance of regulatory, accreditation, or other quality requirements. Most importantly, supervisors measure the effectiveness of professional development by the achievement of desired individual child outcomes as these are assessed in the operation of the program.*CFOC3 Std. 1.4.4.1*

3. **Probation and Termination:** When a staff member does not meet minimum competency, that staff member is placed on probation.

TITLE/NAME OF STAFF MEMBER

meets with the staff member to design a corrective action plan with specific evaluation measures and time lines and help to enable the staff member to meet the requirements. Failure to achieve the specified competencies at the end of the times set in the corrective action plan is grounds for termination of the staff member's involvement with the facility.

G. Grievances: The grievance procedure for this facility is

GRIEVANCE PROCEDURE.

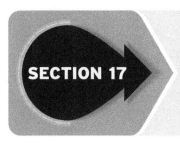

SECTION 17

Design and Maintenance of the Physical Plant and Contents

Rationale

Child care facilities are buildings and grounds where children and families who are unrelated to the teachers/caregivers and adults receive education, care, and support. The children may be infants, toddlers, or preschool- or school-aged children. The building structures and equipment need to be well designed and maintained to enable staff members to protect children, staff members, and family members from injury; prevent disease; and promote the well-being of all.

Required Action/Who Is Responsible/How Communicated

A. Building and Fire Inspections

This facility (building and grounds) meets or exceeds federal, state, and local requirements for building design, physical plant, contents, and maintenance. It is inspected annually by

_____

TITLES OF AGENCY OR INSPECTOR

for compliance with applicable building and fire codes.[CFOC3 Std. 5.1.1.2] The records and findings of these inspections are

_____

LOCATION OF DOCUMENTATION OF DATES AND FINDINGS OF INSPECTIONS.

B. General Cleaning of the Facility

Cleaning of the facility is performed according to guidelines written and monitored by

_____

TITLE/NAME OF STAFF MEMBER.

These guidelines are consistent with the recommended schedule in *CFOC3*. (See Appendix U: Routine Schedule for Cleaning, Sanitizing, and Disinfecting.) Sanitizers and disinfectants are chosen based on the recommendations in *CFOC3* Appendix J. The specific procedures and schedule for cleaning of the facility and grounds is available

_____

WHERE PROCEDURES AND SCHEDULE ARE LOCATED.

The personnel responsible for carrying out general cleaning of the facility are

_____

TITLE/NAME OF STAFF MEMBER OR CONTRACTOR.

In addition, each staff member is responsible for keeping the facility tidy and cleaning up spills when they occur.

C. **Storage and Use of Potentially Toxic Materials**

All potentially toxic materials such as pesticides, toxic cleaning materials, aerosol cans, and poisons will be used according to manufacturer's instructions and under the supervision of

_____

TITLE/NAME OF STAFF MEMBER.

These materials are stored in

_____

LOCATION

away from food and medication and inaccessible to children at all times. In no instance will these materials be used so that children are exposed to any hazard.

D. **Use of Facility and Grounds**

During the hours of program operation, the facility and grounds will not be used for any purpose except the care and education of children and related family services.^{CFOC3 Std. 5.1.1.9}

E. **Facility Design, Space Allocation, and Maintenance**

_____

TITLE(S)/NAME(S) OF STAFF MEMBER(S)

are responsible for review and compliance with the standards in *CFOC3*. These standards address ventilation/heat/cooling/hot water, lighting, noise, electrical service, fire warning systems, water, sewage and garbage, integrated pest management, prevention of exposure to toxic substances, furnishings and finishes, equipment, allocation and occupancy of spaces, toilet/changing areas, sleeping areas, areas for special use, play areas inside and outdoors, and specific requirements for maintenance of all aspects of the facility.^{CFOC3 Stds. 5.1–5.7, 6.1–6.4}

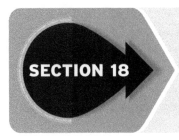

Review and Revision of Policies, Plans, and Procedures

A. Routine Review of Policies

_____
TITLE/NAME OF STAFF MEMBER

will review the applicable policies, plans, and procedures with families, teachers/caregivers, staff members (paid and volunteer), and consultants at the beginning of their involvement with the program and on an annual basis thereafter, as well as whenever policies are changed. Copies of standing policies are always available for family or staff review during the facility's hours of operation in

_____
LOCATION.

Suggestions for updating policies are welcomed from all who are involved in any way with the program.

1. **Review and Acceptance of Policies by Parents/Legal Guardians:** When a child is enrolled in the facility,

_____
TITLE/NAME OF STAFF MEMBER

reviews policies with parents/legal guardians to ensure understanding of the implications for them and their child. Parents/legal guardians will receive a copy of the policies

_____
HOW PARENTS WILL RECEIVE A COPY (EG, AS PART OF A PARENT HANDBOOK)

to read and keep for reference. Parents/legal guardians will sign to indicate that they have read or had the policies explained to them, understand, and agree to abide by these policies.

2. **Review and Acceptance of Policies by Staff Members:** When new staff members (paid or volunteer) are assigned to work in the facility,

_____
TITLE/NAME OF STAFF MEMBER

prepares a list of relevant policies that apply to the new staff member, reviews them, and provides a copy of them

_____
HOW STAFF MEMBERS WILL RECEIVE A COPY (EG, AS PART OF A STAFF HANDBOOK)

for the new staff member to read and retain. New staff members are required to read and agree to comply with the policies that apply to them. They must sign a document that attests to having read, understood, and agreed to abide by the policies and expect disciplinary action for noncompliance.

3. **Revision of Policies:** Revision of policies will involve all administrators, consultants, staff members, and parents/legal guardians, or their representatives (elected by the group being represented), who are affected or have expertise or authority related to the topic addressed by the revision or development of new policies.*CFOC3 Std. 9.2.3.17*

B. Review and Approval of Program Policies (Administrators and Consultants)

_____

SPECIFIC POLICIES APPROVED

_____

NAME, TITLE, AND SIGNATURE OF ADMINISTRATOR OR CONSULTANT WHO APPROVED SPECIFIC POLICIES

_____

DATE

C. Review and Acceptance of Applicable Policies by Staff Members or Parents/Legal Guardians

_____

SPECIFIC POLICIES REVIEWED, UNDERSTOOD, AND AGREED TO

_____

NAME AND SIGNATURE OF STAFF MEMBER OR PARENT/LEGAL GUARDIAN

_____

DATE

D. Acceptance of Occupational Risk by Staff Members: Each staff member (paid or volunteer) is required to review with a supervisor the following acknowledgment of occupational risk and sign the statement to acknowledge and agree to accept the risk:

"I understand there are health risks related to working in child care. These include, but are not limited to, exposure to infectious diseases (including infections that can damage a fetus during a pregnancy), stress, noise, injuries from back strain and biting, skin injury from frequent hand washing, and environmental exposures to art materials and indoor cleaning and disinfecting materials. I have been informed of these risks. I know that I can read the Safety Data Sheets for all products I am required to use. These are located

_____

LOCATION OF THE SAFETY DATA SHEETS.

I agree to follow this facility's written policies and procedures to reduce my exposure to these hazards.

I agree to report any significant health problem I may be having to my supervisor. I understand that I may need to obtain medical treatment for a condition caused by the occupational risks listed herein.

_____

REVIEWED, UNDERSTOOD, AND AGREED TO BY

_____

DATE

Resources

American Academy of Pediatrics, American Public Health Association, National Resource Center for Health and Safety in Child Care and Early Education. *Caring for Our Children: National Health and Safety Performance Standards: Guidelines for Early Care and Education Programs.* 3rd ed. Elk Grove Village, IL: American Academy of Pediatrics; 2011. http://cfoc.nrckids.org. Accessed August 28, 2013

American Academy of Pediatrics. *Managing Infectious Diseases in Child Care and Schools: A Quick Reference Guide.* 3rd ed. Aronson SS, Shope TR, eds. Elk Grove Village, IL: American Academy of Pediatrics; 2013

National Association for the Education of Young Children. *Healthy Young Children: A Manual for Programs.* Aronson SS, ed. 5th ed. Washington, DC: National Association for the Education of Young Children; 2012

Appendix A

Child Care Admission Agreement

_____

NAME OF EARLY CARE AND EDUCATION FACILITY

_____

ADDRESS

_____

PHONE

I, _____

    TITLE/NAME OF STAFF MEMBER

confirm that this child care facility is open

_____

OPERATING DAYS AND HOURS.

Our facility is closed for the following holidays:

_____

HOLIDAYS WHEN FACILITY IS CLOSED.

I have provided, and you _____ have reviewed, accepted, and received a copy of,

                              PARENT/LEGAL GUARDIAN

the following procedures: (Check each as it is reviewed.)

_____ Payment of fees/deposits, late fees/refunds

_____ Drop-off and pickup and daily sign-in/sign-out

_____ Authorized individuals who may pick up my child(ren) and their responsibility to maintain current contact information

_____ Late pickup, nonattendance

_____ Contact of designated individuals in an emergency

_____ Passenger and pedestrian safety

_____ Family member access to the facility whenever the child is in care

_____ Exchange of information about the child with staff members, consultants, and the child's other health care, education, and social service professionals

_____ Content and confidentiality of records, release of information

_____ Infant sleeping practices (for children younger than 12 months)

_____ Documentation of routine health assessments, including immunizations and screening tests, and any conditions that require special accommodations for daily or emergency health or behavioral or developmental support for the child

_____ Inclusion/exclusion for illness

_____ Required clothing for messy activities, outdoor play, and diapering or toileting accidents

_____ Expected family involvement in the child care program

I, _____
PARENT'S NAME

The parent/legal guardian of

_____
CHILD

agree to the following: (Initial all that apply.)

_____ Pay fee per day/week/month on _____
                                              DAY/DATE OF MONTH.

_____ The late payment fee is $ _____ .

_____ Late pickup fee for _____ is $ _____ .
                              MINUTES LATE

_____ Volunteer to work _____ hours a week with the program.
                            HOURS

_____ Comply with the program's policies and procedures.

_____ Obtain a special care plan from my child's health care professional(s) if my child requires any type of care other than what typical children of my child's age usually need.

_____ Provide this special care plan prior to my child's entry/reentry to care that specifies any emergency procedures, medications, or equipment that my child requires.

_____ Review this special care plan with my child's health care professional(s) each time my child receives health care services and ask to have the plan updated as needed.

_____ Whenever the special care plan is updated, provide a copy of the updated plan to the director of this child care program.

_____ Services to be provided as part of the child care fee (eg, transportation, meals) are

_____

_____

_____ Child's planned arrival time _____ Child's planned departure time _____ .

_____ Obtain routine health assessments (checkups, including immunizations) for my child according to the current schedule recommended by the American Academy of Pediatrics.

_____ Notify _____
when my child is scheduled for routine health visits, and obtain a form to complete and return.

_____ Follow up on any medical, dental, or developmental needs of my child identified by my child's health care professional or by staff members of the child care program.

_____ Complete a daily sign-in/sign-out form, and stay until my child's teacher/caregiver welcomes my child and talks with me about plans for the day.

_____ Discuss with my child's teacher/caregiver _____ in advance how to
                                                    AMOUNT OF TIME
celebrate my child's birthday and any special customs for our family related to holiday celebrations.

_____ Notify staff members when my child is ill or any family member has a contagious disease.

_____ Complete medication forms and comply with medication administration procedures when requesting medication administration while my child is in the program.

_____ Provide program staff with _____
necessary for my child's care.   EG, LINENS, FULL CHANGE OF CLOTHING INCLUDING SHOES, TOOTHBRUSH

_____ Provide current information about how to contact me in an emergency situation, which I will update when changes occur and verify at least every 6 months.

_____ Agree to discuss with

_____
TITLE/NAME OF STAFF MEMBER

any concerns related to program operations.

_____ Provide the names and signed and dated photographs of designated persons to whom child may be released for facility records, understanding that these individuals will need to confirm their identity with a photo ID and signature that matches the photo and signature kept in facility records.

_____ Allow my child to be photographed or provide a current picture of my child for staff to carry whenever children are taken off-site or to post in my child's classroom for identification.

_____
PARENT/LEGAL GUARDIAN SIGNATURE   DATE

Note to program administrators: This agreement should be reviewed by legal counsel for your facility.
This is a contract. Many contracts for other types of services include more information than present on this form.

Appendix B

Application for Child Care Services/Enrollment Information

LEGAL NAME OF CHILD | BIRTH DATE | MALE/FEMALE

ADDRESS

CITY | STATE | ZIP CODE

PARENT/LEGAL GUARDIAN #1 | RELATIONSHIP

HOME ADDRESS

WORK ADDRESS

PHONE: HOME | CELL | BUSINESS

BUSINESS HOURS

E-MAIL

PARENT/LEGAL GUARDIAN #2 | RELATIONSHIP

HOME ADDRESS (IF DIFFERENT FROM ABOVE)

WORK ADDRESS

PHONE: HOME | CELL | BUSINESS

BUSINESS HOURS

E-MAIL

DAYS/HOURS WHEN CARE IS NEEDED | REASON FOR ENTRY INTO CHILD CARE

TRANSPORTATION ARRANGEMENT TO AND FROM PROGRAM

....

COMPOSITION OF FAMILY

_____

PARENT/LEGAL GUARDIAN'S FORMAL EDUCATION   (#1) HIGHEST GRADE COMPLETED   (#2) HIGHEST GRADE COMPLETED

_____

LANGUAGE(S) SPOKEN AT HOME

_____

ANY PREVIOUS CHILD CARE EXPERIENCE

Our program does not exclude children with special needs if we can provide a safe environment. The following information is requested to help us plan care for your child:

_____

SPECIAL NEEDS OF PARENTS (EG, INABILITY TO CLIMB STAIRS, DIFFICULTY LIFTING CHILD)

Disability or special needs of child (eg, medications, treatments, allergies, food intolerance, conditions, behaviors) ☐ No ☐ Yes *(Complete special care plan and Authorization for Release of Information forms.)*

_____

USUAL EATING SCHEDULE

_____

FOODS CHILD LIKES   DISLIKES

_____

ELIMINATION PATTERNS (TOILETING/DIAPERING)

_____

THINGS THAT COMFORT CHILD   SCARE CHILD

_____

CULTURAL HABITS/HOME ISSUES THAT MAY AFFECT CHILD'S BEHAVIOR

What is the relationship of the child to the people listed on the Child Care Admission Agreement who are authorized to pick up this child from child care?

_____

NAME AND RELATIONSHIP   NAME AND RELATIONSHIP

_____

NAME AND RELATIONSHIP   NAME AND RELATIONSHIP

_____

WHO WILL CARE FOR THE CHILD WHEN THE CHILD IS TOO ILL TO BE IN THE PROGRAM *(Complete the Emergency Contact and Pickup Information form.)*

_____

PARENT/LEGAL GUARDIAN'S SIGNATURE   DATE

_____

ENROLLMENT DATE

Appendix C

Child Health Assessment

Parent/legal guardian and teachers/child care providers fill in this part.

CHILD'S NAME (LAST)	(FIRST)	PARENT/GUARDIAN
DATE OF BIRTH	HOME PHONE	ADDRESS
CHILD CARE FACILITY NAME		
FACILITY PHONE	COUNTY	WORK PHONE

To parents: Be sure to sign a consent form for your child's teachers/caregivers and one for your child's health care professional to share information about your child's health with one another.

This facility requires that children who are enrolled in a group care setting have received age-appropriate preventive health services, including screenings and immunizations that meet the current recommendations of the American Academy of Pediatrics. This schedule is available on the Internet at http://pediatrics.aappublications.org/content/suppl/2007/12/03/120.6.1376.DC1/Preventive_Health_Care_Chart.pdf.

HEALTH HISTORY AND MEDICAL INFORMATION PERTINENT TO ROUTINE CHILD CARE AND EMERGENCIES (DESCRIBE, IF ANY)	DATE OF MOST RECENT WELL-CHILD EXAM
☐ NONE	_____ This form may be updated (instead of completing a new form) at each checkup visit by the child's health care professional with dated, initialed notes or by attaching a printout of an electronic medical record note.
ALLERGIES TO FOOD OR MEDICINE (DESCRIBE IF ANY) ☐ NONE	

Parents may write immunization dates; health professionals should verify and complete all data.

LENGTH/HEIGHT	WEIGHT	BMI	BLOOD PRESSURE
_____, % _____	_____, % _____	_____, % _____	(Beginning at age 3)
PHYSICAL EXAMINATION	**✓+ NORMAL**		**IF ABNORMAL—COMMENTS**
HEAD/EARS/EYES/NOSE/THROAT		
TEETH		
CARDIORESPIRATORY		
ABDOMEN/GI		
GENITALIA/BREASTS		
EXTREMITIES/JOINT/BACK/CHEST		
SKIN/LYMPH NODES		
NEUROLOGIC & DEVELOPMENTAL		

IMMUNIZATIONS	DATE	DATE	DATE	DATE	DATE	COMMENTS
DTaP, Tdap						
POLIO						
HIB						
HEP B						
MMR						
VARICELLA						
PNEUMOCOCCAL						
ROTAVIRUS						
INFLUENZA						
HEPATITIS A						
HPV						
MENINGOCOCCAL						
OTHER						

SCREENING TESTS	DATE TEST DONE	NOTE HERE IF RESULTS ARE PENDING OR ABNORMAL
LEAD		
ANEMIA (HGB/HCT)		
BEHAVIOR		
LIPID RISK		
HEARING (subjective until age 4)		
VISION (subjective until age 3)		
PROFESSIONAL DENTAL EXAM		NAME OF CHILD'S DENTIST

HEALTH PROBLEMS OR SPECIAL NEEDS, RECOMMENDED TREATMENT/MEDICATIONS/SPECIAL CARE (ATTACH ADDITIONAL SHEETS IF NECESSARY)

☐ NONE   NEXT APPOINTMENT—MONTH/YEAR:

PRINT HEALTH CARE PROFESSIONAL NAME (PEDIATRICIAN, FAMILY PRACTICE PHYSICIAN, OR PEDIATRIC/FAMILY PRACTICE NURSE PRACTITIONER)	SIGNATURE OF PHYSICIAN OR NURSE PRACTITIONER	
ADDRESS		
	PHONE	LICENSE NUMBER	DATE FORM COMPLETED OR UPDATED

Appendix D

Recommendations for Preventive Pediatric Health Care

American Academy of Pediatrics
DEDICATED TO THE HEALTH OF ALL CHILDREN®

Recommendations for Preventive Pediatric Health Care

Bright Futures — Prevention and health promotion for infants, children, adolescents, and their families™

Each child and family is unique; therefore, these **Recommendations for Preventive Pediatric Health Care** are designed for the care of children who are receiving competent parenting, have no manifestations of any important health problems, and are growing and developing in satisfactory fashion. **Additional visits may become necessary** if circumstances suggest variations from normal.

Developmental, psychosocial, and chronic disease issues for children and adolescents may require frequent counseling and treatment visits separate from preventive care visits.

These guidelines represent a consensus by the American Academy of Pediatrics (AAP) and Bright Futures. The AAP continues to emphasize the great importance of **continuity of care** in comprehensive health supervision and the need to avoid fragmentation of care.

The recommendations in this statement do not indicate an exclusive course of treatment or standard of medical care. Variations, taking into account individual circumstances, may be appropriate.

Copyright © 2008 by the American Academy of Pediatrics.

No part of this statement may be reproduced in any form or by any means without prior written permission from the American Academy of Pediatrics except for one copy for personal use.

Schedule

Age groups: **INFANCY** — **EARLY CHILDHOOD** — **MIDDLE CHILDHOOD** — **ADOLESCENCE**

Age columns: Prenatal, Newborn, 3–5 d, By 1 mo, 2 mo, 4 mo, 6 mo, 9 mo, 12 m, 15 m, 18 m, 24 m, 30 mo, 3 y, 4 y, 5 y, 6 y, 7 y, 8 y, 9 y, 10 y, 11 y, 12 y, 13 y, 14 y, 15 y, 16 y, 17 y, 18 y, 19 y, 20 y, 21 y

HISTORY
- Initial/interval

MEASUREMENTS
- Length/height and weight
- Head circumference
- Weight for length
- Body mass index
- Blood pressure

SENSORY SCREENING
- Vision
- Hearing

DEVELOPMENTAL/BEHAVIORAL ASSESSMENT
- Developmental screening
- Autism screening
- Developmental surveillance
- Psychosocial/behavioral assessment
- Alcohol and drug use assessment

PHYSICAL EXAMINATION

PROCEDURES
- Newborn metabolic/hemoglobin screening
- Immunization
- Hematocrit or hemoglobin
- Lead screening
- Tuberculin test
- Dyslipidemia screening
- STI screening
- Cervical dysplasia screening

ORAL HEALTH

ANTICIPATORY GUIDANCE

Legend

● = to be performed   ★ = risk assessment to be performed, with appropriate action to follow, if positive   ●——→ = range during which a service may be provided, with the symbol indicating the preferred age

Footnotes

a. If a child comes under care for the first time at any point on the schedule, or if any items are not accomplished at the suggested age, the schedule should be brought up to date at the earliest possible time.

b. A prenatal visit is recommended for parents who are at high risk, for first-time parents, and for those who request a conference. The prenatal visit should include anticipatory guidance, pertinent medical history, and a discussion of benefits of breastfeeding and planned method of feeding per AAP statement "The Prenatal Visit" (2001). [URL: http://aappolicy.aappublications.org/cgi/content/full/pediatrics;107/6/1456].

c. Every infant should have a newborn evaluation after birth, breastfeeding encouraged, and instruction and support offered. Every infant should have an evaluation within 3 to 5 days of birth and within 48 to 72 hours after discharge from the hospital to include evaluation for feeding and jaundice. Breastfeeding infants should receive formal breastfeeding evaluation, encouragement, and instruction as recommended in AAP statement "Breastfeeding and the Use of Human Milk" (2005) [URL: http://aappolicy.aappublications.org/cgi/content/full/pediatrics;115/2/496]. For newborns discharged in less than 48 hours after delivery, the infant must be examined within 48 hours of discharge per AAP statement "Hospital Stay for Healthy Term Newborns" (2004) [URL: http://aappolicy.aappublications.org/cgi/content/full/pediatrics;113/5/1434].

d. Blood pressure measurement in infants and children with specific risk conditions should be performed at visits before age 3 years.

e. If the patient is uncooperative, rescreen within 6 months per AAP statement "Eye Examination and Vision Screening in Infants, Children, and Young Adults" (1996) [URL: http://aappolicy.aappublications.org/cgi/reprint/pediatrics;98/1/153.pdf].

f. All newborns should be screened per AAP statement "Year 2000 Position Statement: Principles and Guidelines for Early Hearing Detection and Intervention Programs" (2000) [URL: http://aappolicy.aappublications.org/cgi/content/full/pediatrics;106/4/798], Joint Committee on Infant Hearing, "Year 2007 position statement: principles and guidelines for early hearing detection and intervention programs. Pediatrics. 2007;120;898-921.

g. AAP Council on Children With Disabilities, AAP Section on Developmental Behavioral Pediatrics, AAP Bright Futures Steering Committee, AAP Medical Home Initiatives for Children With Special Needs Project Advisory Committee. Identifying infants and young children with developmental disorders in the medical home: an algorithm for developmental surveillance and screening. Pediatrics. 2006;118:405-420. [URL: http://aappolicy.aappublications.org/cgi/content/full/pediatrics;118/1/405].

h. Gupta VB, Hyman SL, Johnson CP, et al. Identifying children with autism early? Pediatrics. 2007;119:152-153 [URL: http://pediatrics.aappublications.org/cgi/content/full/119/1/152].

i. At each visit, age-appropriate physical examination is essential, with infant totally unclothed, older child undressed and suitably draped.

j. These may be modified, depending on entry point into schedule and individual need.

k. Newborn metabolic and hemoglobin screening should be done according to state law. Results should be reviewed at visits and appropriate retesting or referral done as needed.

l. Schedules per the Committee on Infectious Diseases, published annually in the January issue of Pediatrics. Every visit should be an opportunity to update and complete a child's immunizations.

m. See AAP Pediatric Nutrition Handbook, 6th Edition (2003) for a discussion of universal and selective screening options. See also Recommendations to prevent and control iron deficiency in the United States. MMWR Recomm Rep. 1998;47(RR-3):1–36.

n. For children at risk of lead exposure, consult the AAP statement "Lead Exposure in Children: Prevention, Detection, and Management" (2005) [URL: http://aappolicy.aappublications.org/cgi/content/full/pediatrics;116/4/1036]. Additionally, screening should be done in accordance with state law where applicable.

o. Perform risk assessments or screens as appropriate, based on universal screening requirements for patients with Medicaid or in high-prevalence areas.

p. Tuberculosis testing per recommendations of the Committee on Infectious Diseases, published in the current edition of Red Book: Report of the Committee on Infectious Diseases. Testing should be done on recognition of high-risk factors.

q. "Third Report of the National Cholesterol Education Program (NCEP) Expert Panel on Detection, Evaluation, and Treatment of High Blood Cholesterol in Adults (Adult Treatment Panel III) Final Report" (2002) [URL: http://circ.ahajournals.org/cgi/content/full/106/25/3143] and "The Expert Committee Recommendations on the Assessment, Prevention, and Treatment of Child and Adolescent Overweight and Obesity," Supplement to Pediatrics. In press.

r. All sexually active patients should be screened for sexually transmitted infections (STIs).

s. All sexually active girls should have screening for cervical dysplasia as part of a pelvic examination beginning within 3 years of onset of sexual activity or age 21 (whichever comes first).

t. Referral to dental home, if available. Otherwise, administer oral health risk assessment. If the primary water source is deficient in fluoride, consider oral fluoride supplementation. At the visits for 3 years and 6 years of age, it should be determined whether the patient has a dental home. If the patient does not have a dental home, a referral should be made to one. If the primary water source is deficient in fluoride, consider oral fluoride supplementation.

u. Refer to the specific guidance by age as listed in Bright Futures Guidelines. (Hagan JF, Shaw JS, Duncan PM, eds. Bright Futures: Guidelines for Health Supervision of Infants, Children, and Adolescents, 3rd ed. Elk Grove Village, IL: American Academy of Pediatrics; 2008.)

Appendix E

Refusal to Vaccinate

_____

CHILD'S/ADULT WORKER'S NAME

_____

CHILD'S PARENT'S/GUARDIAN'S NAME

I have had the opportunity to discuss the recommended vaccines and my refusal with my/my child's doctor or nurse, who has answered all of my questions about the recommended vaccine(s). I have had the opportunity to review a list of reasons for vaccinating, possible health consequences of non-vaccination, and possible side effects of each vaccine on the Web site of the Centers for Disease Control and Prevention at www.cdc.gov/vaccines/pubs/vis/default.htm.

I still decline the following nationally recommended immunizations:

Name of Vaccine	Check if Recommended for Age and Risk	Declined or Delayed; Initials and Date
Hepatitis B		
Diphtheria, tetanus, acellular pertussis (DTaP or Tdap)		
Diphtheria, tetanus (DT or Td)		
Haemophilus influenzae type b (Hib)		
Pneumococcal conjugate or polysaccharide		
Inactivated poliovirus (IPV)		
Measles-mumps-rubella (MMR)		
Varicella (chickenpox)		
Influenza (flu)		
Meningococcal conjugate or polysaccharide		
Hepatitis A		
Rotavirus		
Human papillomavirus (HPV)		
Other		

I understand the following:

- The purpose of and the need for the recommended vaccine(s).

- The risks and benefits of the recommended vaccine(s).

- That some vaccine-preventable diseases are common in other countries and that unvaccinated people could easily get one of these diseases while traveling or from a traveler who comes to anyplace in my community.

- Without receiving the vaccine(s) according to the medically accepted schedule, the consequences may include getting the disease that could increase the risk of certain types of cancer, pneumonia, illness requiring hospitalization, death, brain damage, paralysis, meningitis, seizures, and deafness, as well as other severe and permanent effects.

- Spreading the disease to others (including those too young to be vaccinated or those with immune problems), possibly requiring staying at home for a prolonged time.

I agree to tell all health care and all education professionals in all settings what vaccines I/my child have/has not received. Lacking immunization may require isolation or immediate medical evaluation and tests that might not be necessary if the vaccines had been given.

I know that I may revisit this issue with my (child's) doctor or nurse at any time and that I may change my mind and accept vaccination any time in the future.

I acknowledge that I have read this document in its entirety and fully understand it.

_____   _____
ADULT WORKER OR PARENT/GUARDIAN SIGNATURE   DATE

_____
WITNESS NAME (PRINT)

_____   _____
WITNESS SIGNATURE   DATE

Reliable Immunization Resources for Educators and Parents/Legal Guardians

Web sites

1. **American Academy of Pediatrics (AAP) Childhood Immunization Support Program (CISP)**

   Information for providers and parents.

   www.aap.org/immunization

   www2.aap.org/immunization/pediatricians/refusaltovaccinate.html

2. **Immunization Action Coalition (IAC)**

   The IAC works to increase immunization rates by creating and distributing educational materials for health professionals and the public that enhance the delivery of safe and effective immunization services. The IAC "Unprotected People Reports" are case reports, personal testimonies, and newspaper and journal articles about people who have suffered or died from vaccine-preventable diseases.

   www.immunize.org/reports

3. **Centers for Disease Control and Prevention (CDC) National Immunization Program**

   Information about vaccine safety. Provide possible health consequences of non-vaccination and possible side effects of each vaccine.

   www.cdc.gov/vaccines/parents/index.html

   www.cdc.gov/vaccines/pubs/vis/default.htm

   www.cdc.gov/vaccines/hcp.htm

4. **National Network for Immunization Information (NNii)**

   Includes information to help answer patients' questions and provide the facts about immunizations.

   www.immunizationinfo.org/professionals

   www.immunizationinfo.org/parents

5. **Vaccine Education Center at Children's Hospital of Philadelphia**

   Information for parents includes "Vaccine Safety FAQs" and "A Look at Each Vaccine."

   www.vaccine.chop.edu

6. **Why Immunize?**

   A description of the individual diseases and the benefits expected from vaccination.

   www2.aap.org/immunization/families/faq/whyimmunize.pdf

7. **Institute for Vaccine Safety, Johns Hopkins Bloomberg School of Public Health**

   Provides an independent assessment of vaccines and vaccine safety to help guide decision-makers and educate physicians, the public, and the media about key issues surrounding the safety of vaccines.

   www.vaccinesafety.edu

8. Pennsylvania Immunization Education Program of Pennsylvania Chapter, AAP

Includes answers to common vaccine questions and topics, such as addressing vaccine safety concerns, evaluating anti-vaccine claims, sources of accurate immunization information on the Web, and talking with parents about vaccine safety.

www.paiep.org

9. Immunize Canada

Immunize Canada aims to meet the goal of eliminating vaccine-preventable disease through education, promotion, advocacy, and media relations. It includes resources for parents and providers.

www.immunize.cpha.ca/en/default.aspx

Handout

1. Immunization Action Coalition. Reliable sources of immunization information: where to go to find answers! http://www.immunize.org/catg.d/p4012.pdf. Accessed July 8, 2013

Books

1. Myers MG, Pineda D. *Do Vaccines Cause That?! A Guide for Evaluating Vaccine Safety Concerns.* Galveston, TX: Immunizations for Public Health; 2008

2. Offit PA. *Autism's False Prophets: Bad Science, Risky Medicine, and the Search for a Cure.* New York, NY: Columbia University Press; 2008

3. Offit PA. *Deadly Choices: How the Anti-Vaccine Movement Threatens Us All.* New York, NY: Basic Books; 2011

4. Mnookin S. *The Panic Virus: A True Story of Medicine, Science, and Fear.* New York, NY: Simon and Schuster; 2011

5. Offit PA, Moser CA. *Vaccines and Your Child: Separating Fact from Fiction.* New York, NY: Columbia University Press; 2011

Appendix F

Staff and Child Emergency Contact and Child Pickup Information

(The information on this form is confidential, to be shared only with written consent of the source of the information.)

CHILD'S/STAFF MEMBER'S LEGAL NAME   BIRTH DATE

CHILD'S/STAFF MEMBER'S USUAL ARRIVAL TIME   USUAL DEPARTURE TIME

IF PART-TIME, WHAT DAYS?

DATE ENROLLED/WORKED IN PROGRAM   OTHER CURRENT ENROLLMENT/WORK ARRANGEMENTS

Contact Information

PARENT/LEGAL GUARDIAN/NEXT OF KIN #1 NAME

RELATIONSHIP

TELEPHONE NUMBERS
                    HOME   CELL   WORK

E-MAIL(S)

LANGUAGE(S) SPOKEN
                    PREFERRED   OTHER LANGUAGES SPOKEN

WORK/SCHOOL NAME OF PARENT/LEGAL GUARDIAN   STUDENT? YES NO

WORK/SCHOOL ADDRESS:NAME OF SUPERVISOR/PRINCIPAL

PARENT/LEGAL GUARDIAN/NEXT OF KIN #2 NAME

RELATIONSHIP

TELEPHONE NUMBERS _____
                              HOME   CELL   WORK

E-MAIL(S)

LANGUAGE(S) SPOKEN _____
                              PREFERRED   OTHER LANGUAGES SPOKEN

WORK/SCHOOL NAME OF PARENT/LEGAL GUARDIAN   STUDENT? YES NO

WORK/SCHOOL ADDRESS

NAME OF SUPERVISOR/PRINCIPAL

Backup Emergency Contacts

(Individuals to whom a child may be released if parent/legal guardian is unavailable or who may be contacted in an emergency for a staff member or for a child.)

EMERGENCY CONTACT #1

RELATIONSHIP

TELEPHONE NUMBERS _____
(CIRCLE ONE TO TRY FIRST.)   HOME   CELL   WORK

E-MAIL(S)

LANGUAGE(S) SPOKEN _____
                              PREFERRED   OTHER LANGUAGES SPOKEN

EMERGENCY CONTACT #2

RELATIONSHIP

TELEPHONE NUMBERS
(CIRCLE ONE TO TRY FIRST.)   HOME   CELL   WORK

E-MAIL(S)

LANGUAGE(S) SPOKEN
                    PREFERRED   OTHER LANGUAGES SPOKEN

Household Members Who Live in the Child's/Staff Member's Home

Name	Relationship	Date of Birth/Age

(Attach extra sheets if needed to list additional household members.)

Child's/Staff Member's Usual Source of Medical Care

NAME

ADDRESS

TELEPHONE NUMBER

Child's/Staff Member's Usual Source of Dental Care

NAME

ADDRESS

TELEPHONE NUMBER

Child's/Staff Member's Health Insurance

NAME OF INSURANCE PLAN   ID #

SUBSCRIBER'S NAME (ON INSURANCE CARD)

Special Conditions, Disabilities, Allergies, or Medical Information for Emergency Situations

Name any concern that might require special care and be sure to complete the Emergency Information Form for Children/Staff Members With Special Needs. Expect and give permission for the center to post the name, photo, and type of health concern the child/staff member has that might require an emergency response, eg, food allergy, severe reaction to insect stings, asthma, blood sugar condition, medication problem.

Transport Arrangement in an Emergency Situation

In an emergency, the program will call 911. Usually, emergency medical services first responders will take sick or

injured children to _____ and adult patients to _____.

NAME OF HOSPITAL .... NAME OF HOSPITAL

Parent/Legal Guardian/Staff Member Consent

As parent/legal guardian/staff member, I give consent for my child/me to receive first aid from facility staff and, if necessary, to be transported to receive emergency care. I understand that I will be responsible for all charges not covered by insurance. The information on this form may be shared with staff members who are responsible for supervision of my child/staff. I understand that I will be asked to sign separate consent forms for medication administration, release of confidential information, field trips, and special program activities.

For child pickup and emergencies: If I am unavailable for a routine or emergency pickup of a child, I give consent for the emergency contact person listed previously **to act on my behalf** until I am available. I understand that a photo ID and interview related to information on this form will be requested by staff members to be sure that the person picking up my child is a person who is listed on this form as a person who is authorized to do so. I agree to review and update this information whenever a change occurs and at least every 6 months.

_____

DATE   PARENT/LEGAL GUARDIAN'S/STAFF MEMBER'S SIGNATURE #1

_____

DATE   PARENT/LEGAL GUARDIAN'S/STAFF MEMBER'S SIGNATURE #2

_____

DATE   EMERGENCY CONTACT PERSON'S SIGNATURE #1

_____

DATE   EMERGENCY CONTACT PERSON'S SIGNATURE #2

Appendix G

···

Special Care Plan Forms

Care Plan for a Child With Special Needs in Child Care   Today's Date _____

Full Name of Child	Birth Date	Child's Present Weight
Parent's/Legal Guardian's Name (Please * first person to contact.)	Cell/Home/Work Phone #	Signature for Consent*
Emergency Contact Person (Name/Relationship)	Cell/Home/Work Phone #	*Consent for health care professional to communicate with my child's teacher/child care provider to discuss information relating to this care plan
Primary Health Care Professional	Emergency Phone #	Authorization for Release of Information Form completed? ☐N/A ☐Yes ☐No
Specialty Provider	Emergency Phone #	Emergency Information Form for Children With Special Needs completed? ☐N/A ☐Yes ☐No
Specialty Provider	Emergency Phone #	Specialty Care Plan(s) completed? ☐N/A ☐Yes ☐No

Allergies   ☐ No   ☐ Yes If yes, please specify.

Medical/Behavioral Concerns

Needed Accommodations (Please describe accommodation and why it is necessary. Attach additional pages if needed to provide complete information.)

Diet/Feeding	Toileting
Classroom Activities	Outdoor or Field Trips
Nap/Sleep	Transportation

Recommended Treatment		
Medications to Be Given at Child Care ☐ No ☐ Yes		If yes, Medication Administration Forms completed? ☐ Yes ☐ No
Specify medications on Medication Administration Forms.		
Medications Given at Home ☐ No ☐ Yes		If yes, please list in additional information section or attach info.
Special Equipment/Medical Supplies ☐ No ☐ Yes		If yes, please list in additional information section or attach info.
Special Staff Training Needs ☐ No ☐ Yes		If yes, please list in additional information section or attach info.
Special Emergency Procedures ☐ No ☐ Yes		If yes, please list in additional information section or attach info.
Other Specialists Working With This Child ☐ No ☐ Yes		If yes, please list and indicate the role(s) of specialists who are working with the child.
Parent/Legal Guardian Signature Acknowledging Review of Above Information		
Additional Information/Comments on Child, Family, or Medical Issues		Additional Information Attached ☐ No ☐ Yes
Health Care Professional's Signature		Health Care Professional's Name Printed

BEHAVIORAL DATA COLLECTION SHEET

This sheet is intended to be used by caregivers to document a child's behavior that is of concern to them. The behavior may warrant evaluation by a health care provider, discussion with parents, and/or consultation with other professionals.

Child's name: _____   Date: _____

1. Describe behavior observed: (See below for some descriptions.)

   _____

2. Behavior noted from: _____ to _____
                         (time)   *(time)*

3. During that time, how often did the child engage in the behavior? (e.g. once, 2-5 times, 6-10 times, 11-25 times, >25 times, >100 times) _____

4. What activity(ies) was the child involved in when the behavior occurred? (e.g. Was the child involved in a task? Was the child alone? Had the child been denied access to a special toy, food, or activity?) _____

5. Where did the behavior occur? _____

6. Who was around the child when the behavior began? List staff, children, parents, others.

   _____

7. Did the behavior seem to occur for no reason? Did it seem affected by changes in the environment?

   _____

8. Did the child sustain any self-injury? Describe. _____

9. Did the child cause property damage or injury to others? Describe. _____

   _____

10. How did caregiver respond to the child's behavior? If others were involved, how did they respond?

    _____

11. What did the child do after caregiver's response? _____

12. Have parents reported any unusual situation or experience the child had since attending child care?

Child Care Facility Name: _____

Name of Teacher/Caregiver (completing this form): _____

Behaviors can include:
- *repetitive, self-stimulating acts*
- *self-injurious behavior (SIB) such as head banging, self-biting, eye-poking, pica (eating non-food items), pulling out own hair*
- *aggression / injury to others*
- *disruption such as throwing things, banging on walls, stripping*
- *agitation such as screaming, pacing, hyperventilating*
- *refusing to eat / speak; acting detached / withdrawn*
- *others*

Check a child's developmental stage before labeling a behavior a problem. For example, it is not unusual for a 12 month old to eat non-food items, nor is it unusual for an 18 month old to throw things. Also, note how regularly the child exhibits the behavior. An isolated behavior is usually not a problem.

S. Bradley, JD, RN,C - PA Chapter American Academy of Pediatrics
reviewed by J. Hampel, PhD and R. Zager, MD

SPECIAL CARE PLAN FOR A CHILD WITH BEHAVIOR CONCERNS

*This sheet is intended to be used by health care providers and other professionals
to formulate a plan of care for children with behavior concerns
that parents and child care providers can agree upon and follow consistently.*

Part A: To be completed by parent/legal guardian.

Child's name: _____   Date of birth: _____

Parent name(s):_____   _____

Phone:_____ Cell: _____ E-Mail: _____

Parent emergency numbers: _____   _____

Child care facility/school name: _____   Phone: _____

Health care provider's name: _____   Phone: _____

Other specialist's name/title: _____   Phone: _____

Part B: To be completed by health care provider, pediatric psychiatrist, child psychologist, or other specialist.

1. Identify/describe behavior concern: _____

2. Possible causes/purposes for this type of behavior: (Circle all that apply.)

    medical condition _____   tension release
    _____(specify)_____
                                                       developmental disorder

    attention-getting mechanism   neurochemical imbalance

    gain access to restricted items/activities   frustration

    escape performance of task   poor self-regulation skills

    psychiatric disorder _____   other: _____
    _____(specify)_____

3. Accommodations needed by this child: _____

    _____

4. List any precipitating factors known to trigger behavior: _____

    _____

5. How should caregiver react when behavior begins? (Circle all that apply.)

    ignore behavior   physical guidance (including hand-over-hand)

    avoid eye contact/conversation   model behavior

    request desired behavior   use diversion/distraction

    use helmet*   use substitution

    use pillow or other device to block self-injurious behavior (SIB)*

    other: _____

    _____

    *directions for use described by health professional in Part D.

6. List any special equipment this child needs: _____

_____

7. List any medications this child receives:

        Name of medication: _____   Name of medication: _____

        Dose: _____   Dose: _____

        When to use: _____   When to use: _____

        Side effects: _____   Side effects: _____

        _____   _____

        Special instructions: _____   Special instructions: _____

        _____   _____

        If the child is to receive medication while in the early education/program, prescription and medication forms will be required.

8. Training staff need to care for this child: _____

_____

9. List any other instructions for teachers/caregivers: _____

_____

Part C: Signatures

Date to review/update this plan: _____

Health care provider's signature: _____ Date: _____

Other specialist's signature: _____ Date: _____

Parent's/Legal Guardian's signature(s): _____ Date: _____

_____ Date: _____

Child care/school director: _____ Date: _____

Primary caregiver/teacher signature: _____ Date: _____

Part D: To be completed by health care provider, pediatric psychiatrist, child psychologist, or other specialist.

Directions for use of helmet, pillow, or other behavior protocol: _____

_____

_____

_____

_____

_____

Updated May 2013 from an original form created by S. Bradley, JD, RN, C - PA Chapter American Academy of Pediatrics reviewed by J. Hampel, PhD and R. Zager, MD
April, 1997

Appendix H

How to Use Special Care Plans

Definition

A *child with special needs* is a child who has or is at increased risk of chronic physical, developmental, behavioral, or emotional conditions and who requires health and related services of a type or amount beyond that required by children generally.

Which Enrolled Children Have a Special Need?

One in 4 children has a special need. Many early education and child care programs enroll children who have behavior concerns or a developmental delay. Some receive services from a specialist. Ideally, the specialist shares techniques the adults in the child's life can use to improve the child's everyday functioning. The sharing of special care plans helps provide better care for any type of special need—asthma, a seizure disorder, a peanut allergy, difficulty handling transitions, dealing with aggressive impulses, or a lag in acquisition of age-appropriate skills. An excellent way to learn more about children with special needs is to complete the online self-learning module from the Early Childhood Education Linkage System (ECELS) called "Caring for Children with Special Needs." Find and use the self-learning module on the ECELS Web site at www.ecels-healthychildcarepa.org by clicking "Professional Development/Training" in the main menu bar, and then selecting "Self-Learning Modules." In addition to the self-learning module, the ECELS Web site has many useful items related to caring for children with special needs.

Who Needs a Care Plan?

Child care staff members should have a special care plan for any child who has an ongoing medical, developmental, or behavioral condition. Care plans should specify daily care, including care for any situations in which the child might require special care, including an emergency. An excellent reference book for teachers/caregivers is the American Academy of Pediatrics (AAP) *Managing Chronic Health Needs in Child Care and Schools: A Quick Reference Guide,* edited by Elaine A. Donoghue, MD, FAAP, and Colleen A. Kraft, MD, FAAP. This book offers policies and procedures necessary to consider in child care and has more than 35 quick reference sheets for specific conditions.

Why Do Early Care and Education Program Staff Members Need Care Plans?

Teachers/caregivers need as much information as possible about the daily and emergency needs of all children. Include a "Care Plan for a Child With Special Needs in Child Care" and a "Special Care Plan for a Child With Behavior Concerns" in your facility's admission packet. This lets parents/legal guardians know what type of information the program needs. Ask parents/legal guardians to give the completed form to the program before the child's first day. The care plan information guides the education of staff members so they can properly care for the child. Every program needs general policies and procedures for medication administration. Each child who needs medication at home or while in the program should have the details specified in the care plan as well. Some children need special diets or adjustment of their activities or the environment. Some require an individual plan for medical and facility emergencies.

Who Is Responsible for the Care Plan?

Every adult involved in the child's care must know and be able to implement the plan. The child's health care professional should complete the care plan. The parent/legal guardian must help the health care professional understand what the child's program must know and the need to provide this information in nonmedical terms. For some children, the parent/legal guardian can complete most of the form. Then the health care professional should review and add any needed information. For a child with a complex condition, parents/legal guardians should schedule an office visit with the health care professional to discuss and complete the form, which will take more time than usually scheduled for a well-child checkup. The sections that apply to a specific child on the care plan are easy to fill out. Some children will have more than one health care professional or specialist who will contribute additional medical or educational information (eg, Individual Family Service Plan, Individual Education Plan).

What Should a Care Plan Include?

The care plan may be very simple or complex depending on the child's needs.

Possible content includes

- Contact information for families and doctors, including important subspecialists
- Medical condition(s) or behavioral concern(s)
- Allergies
- Medication(s)
- Medical procedure(s)
- Special diet
- Special instructions for classroom accommodation, napping, toileting, outdoor activity, or transportation
- Special equipment or supplies
- Special training or instruction staff may need

Completing the Care Plan for Children With Special Needs

A care plan should be updated to note changes in the child's medical condition or routinely whenever the child has a checkup according to the schedule recommended by the AAP. In many states, early education and child care programs use state-provided forms to collect health information about the child. Some of these forms have sections to note medical conditions, behavioral concerns, or medications which the child may require while in care. If the completed form indicates that any of these conditions exist, the early education and child care program should ask that the child's health care professional also complete a care plan. Following are details about parts of the care plan forms:

Child's Present Weight

The child's current weight is important for emergency medical services (EMS) providers to determine medication dosages in an emergency.

Parent's/Legal Guardian's Name

Be sure to put a * by the person you want to be contacted first and that person's work, home, and cell phone numbers.

Signature for Consent

Parents/guardians should be sure to give consent for health care professionals to communicate with early education and child care program staff members about this care plan. The health care professional may have a special form to sign to comply with the confidentiality requirements of the Health Insurance Portability and Accountability Act of 1996 (HIPAA) that covers health professional communications. The HIPAA form specifies exactly what portions of the medical record parents want released. Early education and child care programs are not covered by HIPAA but should have a signed consent to share confidential information with the child's health care professional.

Specialty Provider

Children with chronic medical problems may have one or more specialists. For example, a child with severe asthma may have an allergist or pulmonary specialist who is primarily responsible for medication adjustments or determining when a visit to the emergency department is necessary. For some children, a pediatrician, nurse practitioner, or family doctor might make these decisions without involving a specialist.

Emergency Information Form for Children With Special Needs Completed

The American College of Emergency Physicians and AAP developed a separate form to collect the information needed by EMS and emergency health care professionals to take care of a child who is new to them. It summarizes the child's medical history. The child's health care professional should decide whether a child needs this form, and if so, complete it. (See Appendix I.)

Specialty Care Plan(s) Completed

For some children, a medical specialist or support group for their medical condition may have developed a care plan specific for their condition (eg, asthma, food allergies, seizures). Note whether the parent/legal guardian and health care professional prefer that child care staff members use these care plans. For a child with more than one chronic condition, a specialty care plan might best explain one condition, and the care plan might best explain another.

Needed Accommodations

Some conditions require adjustment of daily routines. For example, Anthony, age 3 years, has milk, nut, and hay allergies and asthma. Accommodations Anthony needs include having his food brought from home and only served to him for all his meals and special snacks for celebrations set aside for him. With a written, signed, and dated consent from the parent/legal guardian, the program should post a written list of his allergies and his photograph everywhere in the facility Anthony might go. Posting a picture of Anthony with a list of his allergies where all adults can see it will help avoid innocent exposures to his allergy triggers by substitutes, volunteers, and visitors. Everyone must be vigilant about hand washing on arrival at the program each morning to avoid inadvertently exposing Anthony to milk or nuts from someone else's breakfast. A nut-free classroom would be best. His teacher/caregiver wears a fanny pack or otherwise has immediate access to emergency medicine (eg, EpiPen), for which there is a prescription on file at the facility. In addition, if Anthony has a prescription for it, the immediately accessible emergency medication should include an inhaler with a spacer at all times. Everyone who is with Anthony during the day needs to recognize the symptoms of a severe allergic reaction and know where to access and how to use an EpiPen as well as an inhaler with a spacer, if necessary. To reduce the risk of a problem for Anthony, the program might plan a field trip to somewhere other than to a farm while Anthony is in the class.

Recommended Treatment

Daily or emergency treatments may be necessary. In our example, Anthony may need to use a nebulizer or an inhaler with a spacer to receive asthma medications. His teacher/caregiver will need to know how to properly assist Anthony with these treatments.

Medications to Be Given at Child Care

The AAP developed a packet of 3 medication administration forms for child care providers to use: Authorization to Give Medicine, to be completed by the parent; Receiving Medication, to be completed by the child care provider accepting the medication; and Medication Log, to be completed by the child care provider giving the medication. This packet is in Appendix X.

Medications Given at Home

Some children receive medication only at home for chronic conditions. In the event of an emergency, teachers/caregivers must be able to tell health care professionals about *all* medications a child receives.

Special Equipment/Medical Supplies

Teachers/caregivers must understand how to use, clean, and store equipment as well as how to obtain and dispose of supplies.

Special Staff Training Needs/Special Emergency Procedures

Teachers/caregivers must understand and be able to demonstrate whatever is needed for the child's condition. This includes any procedures, treatments, medication administration, and use of equipment and medical supplies. Staff members can acquire much of the needed information and some skills by reading materials on the Web sites of the AAP (www.aap.org) and Centers for Disease Control and Prevention (www.cdc.gov) and participating in workshops led by health professionals or using self-learning modules at the Web site of Early Childhood Education Linkage System (www.ecels-healthychildcarepa.org), a program of the Pennsylvania Chapter of the AAP. Some conditions may require hands-on training with health care professionals.

Other Specialists Working With This Child

Some children have a combination of physical, behavioral/emotional, and developmental chronic conditions. Teachers/caregivers need to know about all recommended therapies from psychologists; physical, occupational, and speech therapists; and other specialists.

Parent/Legal Guardian Signature Acknowledging Review of Form/
Health Care Professional's Signature

The child's health care professional and parents/legal guardians must review and acknowledge by their signatures the information that they are giving to the child's teacher/caregiver.

Appendix I

Emergency Information Form for Children With Special Needs

American College of
Emergency Physicians®

American Academy
of Pediatrics

DATE FORM COMPLETED	REVISED	INITIALS
BY WHOM	REVISED	INITIALS

LAST NAME:

NAME:	BIRTH DATE:	NICKNAME:
HOME ADDRESS:	HOME/WORK PHONE:	
PARENT/GUARDIAN:	EMERGENCY CONTACT NAMES & RELATIONSHIP:	
SIGNATURE/CONSENT*:		
PRIMARY LANGUAGE:	PHONE NUMBER(S):	

PHYSICIANS:	
PRIMARY CARE PHYSICIAN:	EMERGENCY PHONE:
	FAX:
CURRENT SPECIALTY PHYSICIAN:	EMERGENCY PHONE:
SPECIALTY:	FAX:
CURRENT SPECIALTY PHYSICIAN:	EMERGENCY PHONE:
SPECIALTY:	FAX:
ANTICIPATED PRIMARY EMERGENCY DEPARTMENT:	PHARMACY:
ANTICIPATED TERTIARY CARE CENTER:	

DIAGNOSES/PAST PROCEDURES/PHYSICAL EXAM:	
1.	BASELINE PHYSICAL FINDINGS:
2.	
3.	BASELINE VITAL SIGNS:
4.	
SYNOPSIS:	BASELINE NEUROLOGICAL STATUS:

*Consent for release of this form to health care providers.

DIAGNOSES/PAST PROCEDURES/PHYSICAL EXAM CONTINUED:	
MEDICATIONS:	**SIGNIFICANT BASELINE ANCILLARY FINDINGS (LAB, X-RAY, ECG):**
1.	
2.	
3.	
4.	**PROSTHESES/APPLIANCES/ADVANCED TECHNOLOGY DEVICES:**
5.	
6.	

MANAGEMENT DATA:

ALLERGIES: MEDICATIONS/FOODS TO BE AVOIDED	AND WHY:
1.	
2.	
3.	

PROCEDURES TO BE AVOIDED	AND WHY:
1.	
2.	
3.	

IMMUNIZATIONS (mm/yy)

Dates					Dates					
DPT					Hep B					
OPV					Varicella					
MMR					TB status					
HIB					Other					

Antibiotic prophylaxis: Indication: Medication and dose:

COMMON PRESENTING PROBLEMS/FINDINGS WITH SPECIFIC SUGGESTED MANAGEMENTS

Problem	Suggested Diagnostic Studies	Treatment Considerations

COMMENTS ON CHILD, FAMILY, OR OTHER SPECIFIC MEDICAL ISSUES:

Physician/Provider Signature: Print Name:

Appendix J

Authorization for Release of Information

I, _____, give permission for
                                    PARENT OR LEGAL GUARDIAN (PRINT)

_____
                                              PROFESSIONAL/FACILITY

to release to _____ the following information:
                                    RECEIVING PROFESSIONAL/AGENCY

_____
                CONCERNS, SCREENINGS, OBSERVATIONS, DIAGNOSES AND TREATMENTS, RECOMMENDATIONS

This consent is voluntary and may be withdrawn by written notice at any time. The information will be used solely to plan and coordinate the care of my child, will be kept confidential, and may only be shared with

_____
                                              TITLE/NAME OF STAFF MEMBER

Child's Legal Name: _____

Address:_____

City: _____State: _____Zip Code: _____

Date of Birth: _____

_____   _____
PARENT/LEGAL GUARDIAN SIGNATURE   DATE

_____   _____
WITNESS SIGNATURE   DATE

_____
STAFF MEMBER TO BE CONTACTED FOR ADDITIONAL INFORMATION

Appendix K

Consent for Child Care Program Special Activities

Name of Facility: _____

Address of Facility: _____

Child's Legal Name: _____

Consent is given for the items initialed as follows:

Walking Trips

☐ Walking trips to the following locations: _____

Motor Vehicle Transportation

☐ Trips by the program in: _____ to the following locations:
                                                 VEHICLE

_____

_____

☐ Daily transportation by the program in: _____
                                                                    VEHICLE

from: _____ to: _____
                       LOCATION   LOCATION

Children will be restrained during vehicular transport by use of: _____

Special needs of the child during transport: _____

Swimming

☐ Swimming or wading at: _____
                                                        LOCATION

Other Activities (eg, homework supervision, trips to neighborhood playgrounds, special trips)

☐ _____

Parent/Legal Guardian's Name (Print): _____

Parent/Legal Guardian's Signature: _____ Date: _____

(See separate consent forms for emergency care, medication administration, and special dental, dietary, or other needs.)

Appendix L

Family/Teacher–Caregiver Information Exchange Form

Week of _____		Eating			Sleeping			Mood/ Behavior	Stool	Urine	Other
		Normal	Less	More	Normal	Less	More		# of times	# of times	Symptoms of illness, family issues
MON	At Home										
	Child Care am										
	Child Care pm										
TUES	At Home										
	Child Care am										
	Child Care pm										
WED	At Home										
	Child Care am										
	Child Care pm										
THUR	At Home										
	Child Care am										
	Child Care pm										
FRI	At Home										
	Child Care am										
	Child Care pm										

Appendix M

Instructions for Daily Health Check

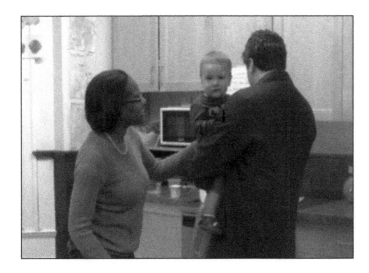

1. Adjust your position to be at the child's level so you can interact with the child even if talking with the parent.

2. Listen to what the family and child tell you and what you see for the following:

    - Complaints about not feeling well.

    - Any suggestion that the child has symptoms of illness or injury.

        - Any symptom or unusual behavior

        - Any bowel problem

        - Any change in usual sleeping/eating/drinking routines

        - When the child most recently ate, used the toilet, had a diaper change, or slept

    - Observed behavior is typical or atypical for time of day and circumstances.

    - Appearance, feel, and look of child's body while touching the child affectionately

        - Skin: pale, flushed, visible rash, unusually warm or cold to the touch, bruises, discomfort when touched.

        - Eyes, nose, mouth: dry or have discharge. Is the child rubbing an eye, nose, or mouth? Is the child sneezing or drooling?

        - Hair: In a lice outbreak, look for nits.

        - Breathing: normal or different, coughing.

Any unusual events, illness in the family, or other experience that might have involved the child.

Appendix N

Enrollment/Attendance/Symptom Record

Group _____

Month _____ **20** ___

For each child, each day: Code top box **+** = present, **O** = scheduled but absent, or **N** = not scheduled. Code bottom box **O** = well or choose from the symptom codes from the bottom of this page.

Legal Name	Age (Months)	Daily Hours in Care	1	2	3	4	5	6	7	8	9	10	11	12	13	14	15	16	17	18	19	20	21	22	23	24	25	26	24	28	29	30	31

SYMPTOM CODES

1 = Asthma, wheezing
2 = Behavior change with no other symptom
3 = Diarrhea
4 = Fever
5 = Headache
6 = Rash
7 = Respiratory (eg, cold, cough, runny nose, earache, sore throat, pinkeye)
8 = Stomachache
9 = Urine problem
10 = Vomiting
11 = Other (Specify on back.)

Appendix O

Daily and Monthly Playground Inspection and Maintenance

For a more comprehensive and updated indoor and outdoor health and safety facility and performance checklist, see "ECELS Health and Safety Checklist 2011 with References" at www.ecels-healthychildcarepa.org (search for "ECELS Health and Safety Checklist"). The "ECELS Health and Safety Checklist" includes references for each item to *Caring for Our Children, Stepping Stones,* and the Infant/Toddler Environment Rating Scale-Revised and Early Childhood Environment Rating Scale-Revised. Another useful checklist is America's Playgrounds Safety Report Card.*CFOC3 Appendix EE* See additional details in the *Public Playground Safety Handbook* at www.cpsc.gov/PageFiles/122149/325.pdf and *Outdoor Home Playground Safety Handbook* at www.cpsc.gov/PageFiles/117306/324.pdf.

Note: The facility inspection and maintenance program should include all recommendations supplied by the manufacturer(s) of play equipment in the facility. Add these recommendations to the items in the checklist in daily, monthly, and biannual inspections.

NAME OF CENTER OR HOME-BASED PROGRAM   NAME OF STAFF DOING INSPECTION

Daily Playground Inspection

(Enter date.) Circle **Y** once if no problem; circle **Y** and **N** each once if a problem is found and fixed; circle **N** twice if problem found but not fixed.

M	T	W	TH	FRI	HAZARD
DATE	DATE	DATE	DATE	DATE	
Y / N	Y / N	Y / N	Y / N	Y / N	1. The entire playground has adequate drainage and is clean/free of trip hazards and hazardous debris/objects (eg, rocks, tree stumps, sticks, litter).
Y / N	Y / N	Y / N	Y / N	Y / N	2. Use zones are free of all obstacles (minimum 3 feet use zone around toddler equipment; 6 feet around all other play equipment).
Y / N	Y / N	Y / N	Y / N	Y / N	3. Check for and take action to remove or repair unsafe or damaged equipment (ie, broken, worn, loose, or missing parts; rust; peeling paint; splinters; sharp edges; cracks/holes; protruding bolts; noticeable gaps; exposed concrete footers; open S hooks; head entrapment openings in guardrails or between ladder rungs that measure between 3.5 and 9 inches).
Y / N	Y / N	Y / N	Y / N	Y / N	4. Rake loose-fill surfacing in areas where it has been displaced.
Y / N	Y / N	Y / N	Y / N	Y / N	5. Sweep loose-fill surfacing, sand, and other debris off of equipment platforms and solid surfaces (eg, asphalt, unitary rubber).
Y / N	Y / N	Y / N	Y / N	Y / N	6. Height of equipment for age of users, type/depth/area of surfacing in fall zones meets the US Consumer Product Safety Commission and ASTM guidelines (See *Handbook for Public Playground Safety*, 2010, excerpts at the end of this form*).
Y / N	Y / N	Y / N	Y / N	Y / N	7. If water tables are used, change water between groups of children; empty, wash, and sanitize water tables and water toys at end of day and prior to use by other classrooms.
Y / N	Y / N	Y / N	Y / N	Y / N	8. Empty trash cans.
Y / N	Y / N	Y / N	Y / N	Y / N	9. Make sure that portable and fixed play structures more than 30 inches high are spaced at least 9 feet apart.
Y / N	Y / N	Y / N	Y / N	Y / N	10. Other (eg, check for animal excrement, litter).

*Excerpts from the *Handbook for Public Playground Safety*, 2010, US Consumer Product Safety Commission, Washington, DC accessed 7/1/2013 at www.cpsc.gov/PageFiles/122149/325.pdf.

Monthly Playground Inspection

(Enter month.) Circle **Y** once if no problem; circle **Y** and **N** each once if a problem is found and fixed; circle **N** twice if problem found but not fixed.

						HAZARD
MONTH	**MONTH**	**MONTH**	**MONTH**	**MONTH**	**MONTH**	
Y / N	Y / N	Y / N	Y / N	Y / N	Y / N	1. Check for and take action on unsafe or damaged equipment (eg, broken parts, rust/peeling paint, splinters, sharp edges, cracks, protruding bolts, gaps, head entrapments).
Y / N	Y / N	Y / N	Y / N	Y / N	Y / N	2. Check for and tighten or replace loose or missing hardware, caps, or plugs.
Y / N	Y / N	Y / N	Y / N	Y / N	Y / N	3. Verify that elevated surfaces (eg, platforms, ramps) have intact guardrails to prevent falls. Check for and replace all moving parts that show wear.
Y / N	Y / N	Y / N	Y / N	Y / N	Y / N	4. Rake loose-fill surfacing to ensure that it is at its proper depth in all areas of use zones.
Y / N	Y / N	Y / N	Y / N	Y / N	Y / N	5. Check all vegetation; clear out hazardous or poisonous weeds; prune dead branches in bushes or trees.

Manufacturers' Specification*

EQUIPMENT	LOCATION	INTENDED AGE OF USERS	TYPE & DEPTH OF SURFACING	USE ZONE**

*See *Handbook for Public Playground Safety*, 2010, excerpts at the end of this form.
**No. of feet around equipment where there is nothing other than surfacing material.

Corrective Action Plan

Hazard to Be Fixed	Person Responsible	Action Needed to Fix Hazard	Date to Be Completed	Date Completed

Examples of Age-Appropriate Equipment		
Toddler Ages 6–23 months	• Climbing equipment under 32" high • Ramps • Single file stepladders • Slides (See CPSC Handbook, paragraph 5.3.6)	• Spiral slides less than 360 degrees • Spring rockers • Stairways • Swings with full bucket seats

Preschool
Ages 2–5 years
	• Certain climbers
	  (See CPSC Handbook, paragraph 5.3.2)
	• Horizontal ladders less than or equal to 60" high
	  for ages 4 and 5
	• Merry-go-rounds
	• Ramps
	• Rung ladders
	• Single file stepladders
		• Slides (See CPSC Handbook, paragraph 5.3.6)
		• Spiral slides up to 360 degrees
		• Spring rockers
		• Stairways
		• Swings—belt, full bucket seats (2–4 years) & rotating tire

Grade School Ages 5–12 years	• Arch climbers • Chain or cable walks • Freestanding climbing events with flexible parts • Fulcrum seesaws • Ladders—horizontal, rung, & step • Overhead rings (See CPSC Handbook, paragraph 5.3.2.5) • Merry-go-rounds • Ramps	• Ring treks • Slides (See CPSC Handbook, paragraph 5.3.6) • Spiral slides more than one 360-degree turn • Stairways • Swings—belt & rotating tire • Track rides • Vertical sliding poles

(from *CPSC Handbook for Public Playground Safety*, 2010, Table 1: p 8)

Fall Heights

(CPSC *Handbook for Public Playground Safety*, 2010, p 41)

5.3.10   Fall height and use zones not specified elsewhere … the following general recommendations should be applied:

- The fall height of a piece of playground equipment is the distance between the highest designated playing surface and the protective surface beneath it.

- The use zone should extend a minimum of 6 feet in all directions from the perimeter of the equipment.

- The use zones of two stationary pieces of playground equipment that are positioned adjacent to one another may overlap if the adjacent designated play surfaces of each structure are no more than 30 inches above the protective surface and the equipment is at least 6 feet apart.

- If adjacent designated play surfaces on either structure exceed a height of 30 inches, the minimum distance between the structures should be 9 feet.

- Use zones should be free of obstacles.

Surfacing

(CPSC Handbook for Public Playground Safety, 2010, p. 8-10)

2.4.2   Selecting a surfacing material

There are two options available for surfacing public playgrounds: unitary and loose-fill materials. A playground should never be installed without protective surfacing of some type. Concrete, asphalt, or other hard surfaces should never be directly under playground equipment. Grass and dirt are not considered protective surfacing because wear and environmental factors can reduce their shock absorbing effectiveness. Carpeting and mats are also not appropriate unless they are tested to and comply with ASTM F1292. Loose-fill should be avoided for playgrounds intended for toddlers.

Appropriate Surfacing

- Any material tested to ASTM F1292, including unitary surfaces, engineered wood fiber, etc.

- Pea gravel

- Sand

- Shredded/recycled rubber mulch

- Wood mulch (not CCA-treated)

- Wood chips

The U.S. Consumer Product Safety Commission
Washington, D.C. 20207 (2008)

"Never Put Children's Climbing Gyms On Hard Surfaces, Indoors Or Outdoors"

"The U.S. Consumer Product Safety Commission (CPSC) is warning parents and daycare providers that children's… climbing equipment should not be used indoors on wood or cement floors, even if covered with carpet, such as indoor/outdoor, shag or other types of carpet. Carpet does not provide adequate protection to prevent injuries."

Appendix P

Staff Assignments for Active (Large-Muscle) Play

WEEK OF	CLIMBERS	SWINGS	SLIDES	RIDING TOYS	OTHER
MON					
TUES					
WED					
THU					
FRI					

Appendix Q

Refrigerator or Freezer Temperature Log

Refrigeration or Freezer Temperature Log for _____ **(Year)** _____

For each workday, find the date and record the temperature in the first box and initials of the person who checked the temperature in the next box. To make it clear whose initials are on this form, print your name and initials at the bottom of this form. Use extra sheets if needed.

Temperature	Initials

Date	Jan		Feb		Mar		April		May		June		July		Aug		Sept		Oct		Nov		Dec	
1																								
2																								
3																								
4																								
5																								
6																								
7																								
8																								
9																								
10																								
11																								
12																								
13																								
14																								
15																								
16																								
17																								
18																								
19																								
20																								
21																								
22																								
23																								
24																								
25																								
26																								
27																								
28																								
29																								
30																								
31																								

Safe Food Temperatures[CFOC3 Std. 4.8.0.6]

Refrigerators: 41°F or lower

Freezers: 0°F or lower

Initials	Print Legal Name

Appendix R

Using Stored Human Milk

1. Fresh milk is better than frozen milk. Use the oldest milk in the refrigerator or freezer first.

2. The baby may drink the milk cool, at room temperature, or warmed. Infants may demonstrate a preference.

3. It is best to defrost human milk in the refrigerator overnight, by running under warm water, or by setting it in a container of warm water. Studies done on defrosting human milk in a microwave demonstrate that controlling the temperature in a microwave is difficult, causing the milk to heat unevenly. Although microwaving milk decreases bacteria in the milk much like pasteurization does, microwaving also significantly decreases the anti-infective quality of human milk, which may reduce its overall health properties for the infant.

4. Once frozen milk is brought to room temperature, its ability to inhibit bacterial growth is lessened, especially by 24 hours after thawing. Previously frozen human milk that has been thawed for 24 hours should not be left out at room temperature for more than a few (about 3) hours.

5. There is little information on refreezing of thawed human milk. Bacterial growth and loss of antibacterial activity in thawed milk will vary depending on the technique of milk thawing, duration of thaw, and amount of bacteria in milk at the time of expression. At this time, no recommendations can be made on the refreezing of thawed human milk.

6. Once a baby begins sucking on a bottle of expressed human milk, some bacterial contamination occurs in the milk from the baby's mouth. The duration of time the milk can be kept at room temperature once the baby has partially fed from the cup or bottle would theoretically depend on the initial bacterial load in the milk, how long the milk has been thawed, and ambient temperature. There have been no studies done to provide recommendations in this regard. Based on related evidence, it seems reasonable to discard the remaining milk within 1 to 2 hours after the baby is finished feeding.

7. Expressed human milk does not require special handling (ie, universal precautions) as is required for other bodily fluids such as blood. It can be stored in a workplace refrigerator where other workers store food, although it should be labeled with child's legal name and date. Mothers may prefer to store their milk in a personal freezer pack.

8. Uncontaminated human milk naturally contains nonpathogenic bacteria and is important in establishing neonatal intestinal flora. These bacteria are probiotics—they create conditions in the intestine that are unfavorable to the growth of pathogenic organisms. If a mother has breast or nipple pain from what is considered to be a bacterial or yeast infection, there is no evidence that her stored expressed milk needs to be discarded. Human milk that appears stringy, foul, or like it has pus in it should not be fed to the baby.

Milk Storage Guidelines

Location of Storage	Temperature That Should Be Maintained (Check with a thermometer in frequently changed water in a glass.)	Maximum Recommended Storage Duration
Room temperature	60°F–85°F (16°C–29°C)	• 3–4 hours optimal • 6–8 hours acceptable under very clean conditions
Refrigerator	<39°F (4°C)	• 72 hours optimal • 5–8 days under very clean conditions
Freezer	<0°F (-17°C)	• 6 months optimal • 12 months acceptable

Adapted from Academy of Breastfeeding Medicine Protocol Committee. ABM clinical protocol #8: human milk storage information for home use for full-term infants (original protocol March 2004; revision #1 March 2010). *Breastfeeding Med.* 2010;5(3):127–130. http://www.bfmed.org/Media/Files/Protocols/Protocol%208%20-%20English%20revised%202010.pdf. Accessed August 30, 2013

Appendix S

Fact Sheet: Choking Hazards

FACT SHEET: Choking Hazards

American Academy
of Pediatrics

DEDICATED TO THE HEALTH OF ALL CHILDREN™

Pennsylvania Chapter

Children under the age of 4 should not be offered foods that are round, hard, small, thick and sticky, smooth, compressible, dense, or slippery. Caring for Our Children Standard 4.5.0.10

EXAMPLES OF HAZARDOUS FOODS

- hot dogs (food that is the most common cause of choking)
        and other meat sticks, whole or sliced into rounds
- hard candy
- peanuts and other nuts
- seeds
- raw peas, raw carrot rounds
- hard pretzels or chips
- rice cakes
- whole grapes
- popcorn
- spoonfuls of peanut butter
- marshmallows
- chunks of meat larger than
   can be swallowed whole

Remember: Children should be seated and supervised while eating.

EASY WAYS TO MAKE FOODS SAFER

Food	Kind of Change

Hot dog	Substitute a more nutritious food;
	    if hot dogs must be served, cut them in quarters lengthwise,
	    then cut the quarter lengths into small pieces.

Whole grapes	Cut in half lengthwise
Nuts	Chop finely
Raw carrots	Chop finely or cut into thin strips
Peanut butter	Spread thinly on inch sized pieces of cucumber, fruit or bread mix with applesauce and spread thinly on bread
Fish or meat with bones	Carefully remove the bones and cut into small pieces

NON-FOOD CAUSES OF CHOKING CARING FOR OUR CHILDREN STANDARD 6.4.1.2

- latex balloons (the most common cause of non-food item causing choking)
- small objects, toys, and toy parts (per Consumer Product Safety Commission, less than 1.25" in diameter and between 1" and 2.25" deep; some recommend a more stringent limit of keeping objects away from young children that have a diameter of less than 1.75")

American Academy of Pediatrics, American Public Health Association, National Resource Center for Health and Safety in Child Care and Early Education. 2011. *Caring for our children: National health and safety performance standards; Guidelines for early care and education programs*. 3rd Edition. Elk Grove Village, IL: AAP; Washington, DC: American Public Health Association.
STD 4.5.0.10: Foods that Are Choking Hazards; STD 6.4.1.2: Inaccessibility of Toys or Objects to Children Under Three Years of Age.
Online at: http://www.nrckids.org.

ECELS-Healthy Child Care PA; PA Chapter, American Academy of Pediatrics 6/2013
Available at www.ecels-healthychildcarepa.org.

Appendix T

Sun Safety Permission Form

Please provide the following materials and give our staff permission to use the indicated measures to help your child stay safe in the sun while in our care:

I _____
        NAME OF PARENT(S)/LEGAL GUARDIAN(S)

agree to supply the following for my child _____ :
                                            LEGAL NAME OF ENROLLED CHILD

1. Wide-brimmed (±3" brim) hat that shades the face, ears, and neck

2. Child-sized sunglasses, polycarbonate or impact-resistant, labeled with 99% to 100% UV lens protection, or prescription glasses with UV protective coating

3. Broad-spectrum (UVA and UVB), PABA (preferably alcohol) free sunscreen, SPF 15 or greater, that is not an

   aerosol or spray (or participate in our facility's bulk purchase of sunscreen by paying _____ for purchase of
                                                                                            $X.XX

   _____
        BRAND-NAME SUNSCREEN

4. Lip balm with SPF 15 or greater

5. Light-colored, lightweight, tightly woven, long-sleeved shirts and long pants

I give permission for my child to receive applications of sunscreen following the manufacturer's instructions.

I understand that sunscreen will be applied 15 to 30 minutes before going outside and every two (2) hours as recommended by the manufacturer.

_____
PARENT/LEGAL GUARDIAN (PRINT)

_____
PARENT/LEGAL GUARDIAN (SIGNATURE)

_____
FACILITY (EARLY LEARNING OR SCHOOL-AGE PROGRAM)   DATE

Sun Safety Permission Form shall remain in effect unless _____
receives written changes.   TITLE/NAME OF STAFF MEMBER

(A physician's signature should not be required for the use of sunscreen. However, if state regulations require a health care professional's signature on this form, add it here.)

_____
HEALTH CARE PROFESSIONAL (SIGNATURE)   DATE

Appendix U

Routine Schedule for Cleaning, Sanitizing, and Disinfecting

Make copies of this guide to use as a checklist on a periodic (eg, monthly) basis to maintain these routines

Areas		Before Each Use	After Each Use	Daily (At the End of the Day)	Weekly	Monthly	Comments
Food Areas	• Food preparation surfaces	Clean, Sanitize	Clean, Sanitize				Use a sanitizer safe for food contact
	• Eating utensils & dishes		Clean, Sanitize				If washing the dishes and utensils by hand, use a sanitizer safe for food contact as the final step in the process; Use of an automated dishwasher will sanitize
	• Tables & highchair trays	Clean, Sanitize	Clean, Sanitize				
	• Countertops		Clean	Clean, Sanitize			Use a sanitizer safe for food contact
	• Food preparation appliances		Clean	Clean, Sanitize			
	• Mixed use tables	Clean, Sanitize					Before serving food
	• Refrigerator					Clean	
Child Care Areas	• Plastic mouthed toys		Clean	Clean, Sanitize			
	• Pacifiers		Clean	Clean, Sanitize			Reserve for use by only one child; Use dishwasher or boil for one minute
	• Hats			Clean			Clean after each use if head lice present
	• Door & cabinet handles			Clean, Disinfect			
	• Floors			Clean			Sweep or vacuum, then damp mop (consider microfiber damp mop to pick up most particles)
	• Machine washable cloth toys				Clean		Launder
	• Dress-up clothes				Clean		Launder
	• Play activity centers				Clean		
	• Drinking Fountains			Clean, Disinfect			

Routine Schedule for Cleaning, Sanitizing, and Disinfecting, *continued*

Areas		Before Each Use	After Each Use	Daily (At the End of the Day)	Weekly	Monthly	Comments
Child Care Areas, *continued*	• Computer keyboards		Clean, Sanitize				Use sanitizing wipes, do not use spray
	• Phone receivers			Clean			
Toilet & Diapering Areas	• Changing tables		Clean, Disinfect				Clean with detergent, rinse,* disinfect
	• Potty chairs		Clean, Disinfect				
	• Handwashing sinks & faucets			Clean, Disinfect			
	• Countertops			Clean, Disinfect			
	• Toilets			Clean, Disinfect			
	• Diaper pails			Clean, Disinfect			
	• Floors			Clean, Disinfect			Damp mop with a floor cleaner/ disinfectant
Sleeping Areas	• Bedsheets & pillowcases				Clean		Clean before use by another child
	• Cribs, cots, & mats				Clean		Clean before use by another child
	• Blankets					Clean	

*The Pennsylvania Chapter of the American Academy of Pediatrics notes that cleaning diaper-changing surfaces with detergent and rinsing with water is necessary only if there is visible soil on the diaper-changing table after removing the disposable paper on which the child was changed. If the surface has no visible soil, the surface doesn't need to be cleaned before disinfecting it.

Adapted from Academy Academy of Pediatrics, American Public Health Association, National Resource Center for Health and Safety in Child Care and Early Education. *Caring for Our Children: National Health and Safety Performance Standards: Guidelines for Early Care and Education Programs.* 3rd ed. Elk Grove Village, IL: American Academy of Pediatrics; 2011:442–443

Appendix V

Major Occupational Health Hazards

Infectious Diseases and Organisms

General Types of Infectious Diseases

Diarrhea (infectious)

Respiratory tract infection

Specific Infectious Diseases and Organisms

Adenovirus

Astrovirus

Caliciviruses

Campylobacter jejuni/coli

Chickenpox (varicella)

Clostridium difficile

Cytomegalovirus (CMV)

Escherichia coli (STEC)

Giardia intestinalis

Haemophilus influenzae type b (Hib)

Hepatitis A

Hepatitis B

Hepatitis C

Herpes 6

Herpes 7

Herpes simplex

Herpes zoster

Human immunodeficiency virus (HIV)

Impetigo

Influenza and H1N1

Lice

Measles

Meningitis (bacterial, viral)

Meningococcus *(Neisseria meningitidis)*

Mumps

Parvovirus B19

Pertussis

Pinworm

Ringworm

Rotavirus

Rubella

Salmonella organisms

Scabies

Shigella organisms

Staphylococcus aureus

Streptococcus, Group A

Streptococcus pneumoniae

Tuberculosis

Injuries and Noninfecious Diseases

Back injuries

Bites

Dermatitis

Falls

Environmental Exposure

Art materials

Cleaning, sanitizing, and disinfecting solutions

Indoor air pollution

Noise

Odor

Outdoor air pollution

Stress

Fear of liability

Inadequate break time, sick time, and personal days

Inadequate facilities

Inadequate pay

Inadequate recognition

Inadequate training

Insufficient professional recognition

Lack of adequate medical/dental health insurance

Responsibility for children's welfare

Undervaluing of work

Working alone/Isolation

Adapted from Academy Academy of Pediatrics, American Public Health Association, National Resource Center for Health and Safety in Child Care and Early Education. *Caring for Our Children: National Health and Safety Performance Standards: Guidelines for Early Care and Education Programs.* 3rd ed. Elk Grove Village, IL: American Academy of Pediatrics; 2011:426

Appendix W

Child Care Staff Health Assessment^{CFOC3} Std. 1.7.01

Employer should complete this section.

Name of person to be examined: _____

Employer for whom examination is being done: _____

Employer's location: _____ Phone number: _____

Purpose of examination: ☐ preemployment (with conditional offer of employment)

☐ annual reexamination

Type of activity on the job: ☐ lifting, carrying children   ☐ close contact with children   ☐ food preparation

☐ desk work   ☐ driver of vehicles   ☐ facility maintenance

Parts I and II must be completed and signed by a licensed physician or certified registered nurse practitioner.

Based on a review of the medical record, health history, and physical examination, does this person have any of the following conditions or problems that might affect job performance or require accommodation?

Date of examination: _____

Part I: Health Problems   (circle)

Visual acuity less than 20/40 (combined, obtained with lenses if needed)?	yes	no
Decreased hearing (less than 20 dB at 500, 1,000, 2,000, 4,000 Hz)?	yes	no
Respiratory problems (asthma, emphysema, airway allergies, current smoker, other)?	yes	no
Heart, blood pressure, or other cardiovascular problems?	yes	no
Gastrointestinal problems (ulcer, colitis, special dietary requirements, obesity, other)?	yes	no
Endocrine problems (diabetes, thyroid, other)?	yes	no
Emotional disorders or addiction (depression, drug or alcohol dependency, difficulty handling stress, other)?	yes	no
Neurologic problems (epilepsy, Parkinson disease, other)?	yes	no
Musculoskeletal problems (low back pain, neck problems, arthritis, limitations on activity)?	yes	no
Skin problems (eczema, rashes, conditions incompatible with frequent hand washing, other)?	yes	no
Immune system problems (from medication, illness, allergies, susceptibility to infection)?	yes	no
Need for more frequent health visits or sick days than the average person?	yes	no
Dental problems assessed in a dental examination within the past 12 months?	yes	no
Other special medical problem or chronic disease that requires work restrictions or accommodation?	yes	no

Part II: Infectious Disease Status

The following immunizations are due/overdue per recommendations for adults in contact with children. Include those listed as follows and any others currently recommended by the Centers for Disease Control and Prevention at www.cdc.gov/vaccines:

Tdap (once, no matter when the most recent Td was given)   yes   no

MMR (2 doses for persons born after 1989; 1 dose for those born in or after 1957)   yes   no

Polio (OPV or IPV in childhood)   yes   no

Hepatitis B (3-dose series)   yes   no

Varicella (2 doses or had the disease)   yes   no

Influenza   yes   no

Pneumococcal vaccine   yes   no

Other vaccines _____

Female of childbearing age susceptible to CMV or parvovirus who needs counseling about risk?   yes   no

Evaluation of TB status shows a risk for communicable TB?   yes   no

Check test used. ☐ Tuberculin skin test (TST) ☐ Interferon gamma release assay (IGRA) test

Test date _____ Result _____

The results and appropriate follow-up of a tuberculosis (TB) screening, using the TST or IGRA, is required once on entering into the child care field with subsequent TB screening as determined by history of high risk for TB thereafter. Anyone with a previously positive TST or IGRA who has symptoms suggestive of active TB should have a chest x-ray. All newly positive TB skin or blood tests should be followed by x-ray evaluation.

Please attach additional sheets to explain all "yes" answers. Include the plan for follow-up.

MD
DO
CRNP

_____

DATE   SIGNATURE   PRINTED LAST NAME   TITLE

Phone number of licensed physician, physician assistant, or certified registered nurse practitioner:

_____

I have read and understand this information.

_____

DATE   PATIENT'S SIGNATURE

Appendix X

Medication Administration Packet

Authorization to Give Medicine
Page 1—To Be Completed by Parent/Guardian

CHILD'S INFORMATION	
NAME OF FACILITY/SCHOOL	TODAY'S DATE
NAME OF CHILD (FIRST AND LAST)	DATE OF BIRTH
NAME OF MEDICINE	
REASON MEDICINE IS NEEDED DURING SCHOOL HOURS	
DOSE	ROUTE
TIME TO GIVE MEDICINE	
ADDITIONAL INSTRUCTIONS	
DATE TO START MEDICINE	STOP DATE
KNOWN SIDE EFFECTS OF MEDICINE	
PLAN OF MANAGEMENT OF SIDE EFFECTS	
CHILD ALLERGIES	

PRESCRIBERS' INFORMATION	
PRESCRIBING HEALTH PROFESSIONAL'S NAME	PHONE NUMBER

PERMISSION TO GIVE MEDICINE

I hereby give permission for the facility/school to administer medicine as prescribed above.
I also give permission for the teacher/caregiver to contact the prescribing health professional about the administration of this medicine.
I have administered at least one dose of medicine to my child without adverse effects.

PARENT OR GUARDIAN NAME (PRINT)		
PARENT OR GUARDIAN SIGNATURE		
ADDRESS		
HOME PHONE NUMBER	WORK PHONE NUMBER	CELL PHONE NUMBER

Receiving Medication
Page 2—To Be Completed by Teacher/Caregiver

NAME OF CHILD

NAME OF MEDICINE

DATE MEDICINE WAS RECEIVED

_____ /_____ /_____

SAFETY CHECK

☐   1. Child-resistant container.

☐   2. Original prescription or manufacturer's label with the name and strength of the medicine.

☐   3. Name of child on container is correct (first and last names).

☐   4. Current date on prescription/expiration label covers period when medicine is to be given.

☐   5. Name and phone number of licensed health care professional who ordered medicine is on container or on file.

☐   6. Copy of Child Health Record is on file.

☐   7. Instructions are clear for dose, route, and time to give medicine.

☐   8. Instructions are clear for storage (eg, temperature) and medicine has been safely stored.

☐   9. Child has had a previous trial dose.

Y ☐   N ☐   10. Is this a controlled substance? If yes, special storage and log may be needed.

TEACHER/CAREGIVER NAME (PRINT)

TEACHER/CAREGIVER SIGNATURE

Medication Log
Page 3—To Be Completed by Teacher/Caregiver

NAME OF CHILD	WEIGHT OF CHILD

	MONDAY	TUESDAY	WEDNESDAY	THURSDAY	FRIDAY
Medicine					
Date					
Actual time given	AM _____ PM _____	AM _____ PM _____	AM _____ PM _____	AM _____ PM _____	AM _____ PM _____
Dosage/amount					
Route					
Staff signature					

	MONDAY	TUESDAY	WEDNESDAY	THURSDAY	FRIDAY
Medicine					
Date					
Actual time given	AM _____ PM _____	AM _____ PM _____	AM _____ PM _____	AM _____ PM _____	AM _____ PM _____
Dosage/amount					
Route					
Staff signature					

Describe error/problem in detail in a Medical Incident Report. Observations can be noted here.

Date/time	Error/problem/reaction to medication	Action taken	Name of parent/guardian notified and time/date	Teacher/caregiver signature

RETURNED to parent/guardian	Date	Parent/guardian signature	Teacher/caregiver signature

DISPOSED of medicine	Date	Teacher/caregiver signature	Witness signature

MEDICATION INCIDENT REPORT	
DATE OF REPORT	SCHOOL/CENTER
NAME OF PERSON COMPLETING THIS REPORT	
SIGNATURE OF PERSON COMPLETING THIS REPORT	
CHILD'S NAME	
DATE OF BIRTH	CLASSROOM/GRADE
DATE INCIDENT OCCURRED	TIME NOTED
PERSON ADMINISTERING MEDICATION	
PRESCRIBING HEALTH CARE PROVIDER	
NAME OF MEDICATION	
DOSE	SCHEDULED TIME

DESCRIBE THE INCIDENT AND HOW IT OCCURRED (WRONG CHILD, MEDICATION, DOSE, TIME, OR ROUTE?)				
ACTION TAKEN/INTERVENTION				
PARENT/GUARDIAN NOTIFIED?	YES	NO	DATE	TIME
NAME OF THE PARENT/GUARDIAN WHO WAS NOTIFIED				
FOLLOW-UP AND OUTCOME				
ADMINISTRATOR'S SIGNATURE				

Preparing to Give Medication

This is a checklist to use at your child care facility/school to make sure that your program is ready to give medication.

1. Paperwork

☐ Parent authorization to give medications is signed.

☐ Health care professional authorization or instructions are on file.

☐ Child Health Record is on file.

2. Medication checked when received

☐ Properly labeled.

☐ Proper container.

☐ Stored correctly.

☐ Instructions are clear.

☐ Disposal plan is developed.

3. Administering medication

☐ Area is clean and quiet.

☐ Staff is trained.

☐ Hands are washed.

☐ The 5 rights are followed—right child, medication, dose, time, and route.

☐ Child is observed for side effects.

4. Documentation

☐ Medication log is completed fully and in ink.

Reference: Academy Academy of Pediatrics, American Public Health Association, National Resource Center for Health and Safety in Child Care and Early Education. *Caring for Our Children: National Health and Safety Performance Standards: Guidelines for Early Care and Education Programs.* 3rd ed. Elk Grove Village, IL: American Academy of Pediatrics; 2011:474–478

The *Curriculum for Managing Infectious Diseases in Early Education and Child Care Settings* is available for reproduction at www.healthychildcare.org/ HealthyFutures.

Appendix Y

Symptom Record

Name of facility/school: _____

Child's legal name: _____

Date: _____ Symptom(s): _____

When symptom began, how long it lasted, how severe, how often? _____
_____

Any change in child's behavior? _____
_____

Child's temperature: _____ Time taken: _____ (Circle: axillary [armpit], oral, rectal, ear canal, other [specify]) _____

How much and what type of food and fluid did the child take in the past 12 hours?_____
_____

Number of times of urination: _____ and bowel movements: _____

How typical/normal were urine and bowel movements in the past _____ hours? _____
_____

Circle or write in other symptoms:

Cough	Headache	Runny nose	Stomachache	Trouble urinating	Other pain (specify) _____
Diarrhea	Itching	Sore throat	Trouble breathing	Vomiting	_____
Earache	Rash	Stiff neck	Trouble sleeping	Wheezing	_____

Other symptoms: _____

Any medications in the past 12 hours (name, time, dose)? _____

Any exposure to animals, insects, soaps, new foods, or new environments? _____
_____

Exposure to other people who were sick; who and what sickness? _____
_____

Child's other problems that might affect this illness (eg, asthma, allergy, anemia, diabetes, emotional trauma, seizures): _____
_____

What has been done so far? _____
_____

Advice from the child's health care professional: _____

_____

Name of person completing this form: _____

Relationship of person completing this form to the child: _____

Appendix Z

Situations That Require Medical Attention Right Away

In the following boxes, you will find lists of common medical emergencies or urgent situations you may encounter as a child care provider. To prepare for such situations

1. Know how to access emergency medical services (EMS) in your area.

2. Know how to reach your poison center—call Poison Help, the national number that connects with the poison center in your region: 1-800-222-1222.

3. Educate staff members about recognition of an emergency. When in doubt, call EMS.

4. Know how to contact each child's parent/legal guardian and have on file consent from the parent/legal guardian to contact the child's primary health care professional in an emergency.

5. Develop plans for dealing with an emergency for children with special health care needs with their family and primary health care professional.

6. Document what happened and what actions were taken. Share this information verbally and in writing with parents/legal guardians.

7. Determine contingency plans for times when there may be power outages, transportation issues, phone communication problems, etc.

Call emergency medical services (EMS) immediately if

- You believe the child's life is at risk or there is a risk of permanent injury.
- The child is acting strangely, much less alert, or much more withdrawn than usual.
- The child has difficulty breathing or is unable to speak.
- The child's skin or lips look blue, purple, or gray.
- The child has rhythmic jerking of arms and legs and loss of consciousness (seizure).
- The child is unconscious.
- The child is less and less responsive.
- The child has any of the following after a head injury: decrease in level of alertness, confusion, headache, vomiting, irritability, difficulty walking.
- The child has increasing or severe pain anywhere.
- The child has a cut or burn that is large or deep or won't stop bleeding.
- The child is vomiting blood.
- The child has a severe stiff neck, headache, and fever.
- The child is significantly dehydrated (eg, sunken eyes, lethargic, not making tears, not urinating).
- Multiple children are affected by injury or serious illness at the same time.
- When in doubt about whether to call EMS, make the call.
- After you have called EMS, call the child's parent/legal guardian.

Some children may have urgent situations that do not necessarily require ambulance transport but still need medical attention without delay. The following box lists some of these situations. The parent/legal guardian should be informed of the following conditions and the need to get prompt medical attention. If you or the parent/legal guardian cannot reach the physician within one hour, the child should be brought to a hospital.

Get medical attention within one hour for

- Fever* in any age child who looks more than mildly ill
- Fever* in a child younger than 2 months (8 weeks)
- A quickly spreading purple or red rash
- A large volume of blood in stools
- A cut that may require stitches
- Any medical condition specifically outlined in a child's care plan requiring parental notification

---

*Fever is defined as a temperature above 100°F (37.8°C) axillary (in the armpit), above 101°F (38.3°C) orally, or above 102°F (38.9°C) rectally, or as measured by an equivalent method.

Appendix AA

Sample Letter to Families About Exposure to Communicable Disease

Name of Child Care Program: _____

Address of Child Care Program: _____

Telephone Number of Child Care Program: _____

Date: _____

Dear Parent or Legal Guardian:

A child in our program has or is suspected of having: _____

Information about this disease

The disease is spread by: _____

The symptoms are: _____

_____

The disease can be prevented by: _____

_____

_____

What the program is doing: _____

What you can do at home: _____

_____

_____

_____

_____

If your child has any symptoms of this disease, call your doctor to find out what to do. Be sure to tell your doctor about this notice. If you do not have a regular doctor to care for your child, contact your local health department for instructions on how to find a doctor or ask other parents for names of their children's doctors. If you have any questions, please contact:

_____ (   )

TEACHER/CAREGIVER'S NAME   PHONE NUMBER

Appendix BB

First Aid Kit Inventory

ITEM	DATE CHECKED (Restock after each use and inventory monthly.)				
Water (bottled or a source of running water to clean injured areas and to remove visible soil from hands); liquid soap (to remove visible soil); and paper towels (to absorb/dry wet surfaces)					
Alcohol-based hand sanitizer (for hand hygiene where running water is not available)					
Disposable, nonporous gloves (to protect hands from contact with blood or body fluids)					
Sealed packages of antiseptic disposable wipes (to remove soil from hands prior to using hand sanitizer)					
Scissors (to cut tape or dressings)					
Tweezers (to remove splinters or ticks)					
Non-glass digital thermometer (to take temperature)					
Bandage tape (to hold gauze pads or splint in place)					
Sterile gauze pads, wrapped sanitary pads (to clean injured area, soak up body fluids, cover cuts and scrapes)					
Nonstick dressing (to cover abrasions)					
Flexible roller gauze (to hold gauze pad, eye pad, or splint in place)					
Adhesive bandages of different sizes (to cover wounds of children older than 4 years; not for younger children because they are a choking hazard)					
Elastic bandage (to put pressure on a bruised or swollen area, hold cold pack in place)					
Triangular bandage (to support injured arm, hold splint in place)					
Safety pins (to pin triangular bandage)					
Eye dressings: soft eye patch or piece of gauze (to bandage lid closed over scratched eye); alternative: paper cup cut down to make a short cap over injured eye					
Pen/pencil and notepad (to write down information and instructions)					
Plastic bags (to dispose of contaminated items)					

ITEM	DATE CHECKED (Restock after each use and inventory monthly.)				
Cold pack (to control swelling and bleeding from bumps and bruises when away from ice); wrap the cold pack in thin cloth before putting it against skin to avoid cold damage to tissues					
Current nationally recognized pediatric first aid instructions (from the American Academy of Pediatrics or the American Heart Association)					
Poison Help telephone number (1-800-222-1222)					
Small plastic metal splint (to immobilize injured finger if splinting to adjacent finger is not practical)					
Emergency medications for children as specified in special care plans that indicate possible need such as auto-injectable medication for a severe allergy or hypoglycemic reaction (to provide a rapid response to emergency); include in kit or in a fanny pack carried by teacher/caregiver responsible for child					
Whistle (to call attention to location of injured person)					
Flashlight					
Battery-powered radio (to receive instructions for community emergency)					
Initials of person who checked the kit contents					

KEEP KIT ACCESSIBLE TO ADULTS AND INACCESSIBLE TO CHILDREN.

INITIALS	PRINT NAME

Sources: American Academy of Pediatrics, American Public Health Association, National Resource Center for Health and Safety in Child Care. Standard 5.6.0.1: first aid and emergency supplies. In: *Caring for Our Children: National Health and Safety Performance Standards: Guidelines for Early Care and Education Programs*. 3rd ed. Elk Grove Village, IL: American Academy of Pediatrics; 2011:257–258, and American Academy of Pediatrics, National Association of School Nurses. *PedFACTs: Pediatric First Aid for Caregivers and Teachers*. 2nd ed. Burlington, MA: Jones & Bartlett Learning; 2014

Appendix CC

Incident Report Form

Fill in all blanks and boxes that apply.

Name of Program: _____ Phone: _____

Address of Facility: _____

Child's Name: _____ Sex: ☐ M ☐ F Birth Date: ___ / ___ / ___ Incident Date: ___ / ___ / ___

Time of Incident: ____ : ____ am/pm Witnesses: _____

Name of Parent/Legal Guardian Notified: _____ Notified by: _____ Time Notified: ____ : ____ am/pm

EMS (911) or Other Medical Professional ☐ Not notified ☐ Notified Time Notified: ___ : ____ am/pm

Location Where Incident Occurred: ☐ Playground ☐ Classroom ☐ Bathroom ☐ Hall ☐ Kitchen ☐ Doorway ☐ Gym

☐ Office ☐ Dining Room ☐ Stairway ☐ Unknown ☐ Other (specify): _____

Equipment/Product Involved: ☐ Climber ☐ Slide ☐ Swing ☐ Playground Surface ☐ Sandbox

☐ Trike/Bike ☐ Hand Toy (specify): _____

☐ Other Equipment (specify): _____

Cause of Injury: Describe: _____

☐ Fall to Surface; Estimated Height of Fall_____feet; Type of Surface: _____

☐ Fall from Running or Tripping ☐ Bitten by Child ☐ Motor Vehicle ☐ Hit or Pushed by Child

☐ Injured by Object ☐ Eating or Choking ☐ Insect Sting/Bite ☐ Animal Bite

☐ Exposure to Cold ☐ Other (specify): _____

Parts of Body Injured: ☐ Eye ☐ Ear ☐ Nose ☐ Mouth ☐ Tooth ☐ Part of Face ☐ Part of Head

☐ Neck ☐ Arm/Wrist/Hand ☐ Leg/Ankle/Foot ☐ Trunk

☐ Other (specify): _____

First Aid Given at the Facility (eg, comfort, pressure, elevation, cold pack, washing, bandage): _____

_____

Treatment Provided by: _____

☐ No doctor's or dentist's treatment required

☐ Treated as an outpatient (eg, office or emergency room)

☐ Hospitalized (overnight) # of days: _____

Number of Days of Limited Activity From This Incident: _____ Follow-up Plan for Care of the Child: _____

_____

Corrective Action Needed to Prevent Reoccurrence: _____

Name of Official/Agency Notified: _____

_____ _____
SIGNATURE OF STAFF MEMBER   DATE

_____ _____
SIGNATURE OF PARENT/LEGAL GUARDIAN   DATE

Copies: 1) Child's folder. 2) Parent. 3) Injury log file.

Appendix DD

Child Care Initial Rapid Damage Assessment

In the aftermath of a disaster, as soon as it is safe to do so, it is imperative to communicate the condition of your facility as well as status of your program with your local Child Care Licensing/Regulatory Compliance Office as soon as possible but no later than 2 days after the incident. Remember, safety comes first! In an event of an emergency, call 911. Make sure staff and children are safe.

The Child Care Initial Rapid Damage Assessment tool was created to standardize the initial rapid damage assessment of the child care community and to be better able to efficiently and effectively respond to situations by providing appropriate assistance and information to families, child care facilities, regulatory agencies, emergency management agencies, and the community.

Objectives of the Child Care Initial Rapid Damage Assessment

- To rapidly assess overall losses to child care facilities

- To rapidly assess interruptions in services provided by child care programs

- To rapidly assess the number of children and staff impacted by the disaster

- To determine the overall operational capability and capacity of the child care community immediately after a disaster

- To inform emergency management officials and community decision makers of the damages sustained by the child care community

- To record available and/or needed resources to support the response and recovery of the child care community

---

Notes:

Reviews and/or updates to Emergency Preparedness Plans should be done within a 1-year period from the date the plan was written, updated, or reviewed.

- Make sure all reviews and updates to the Emergency Preparedness Plan are documented and dated. Keep a dated record of all changes made to the plan.

- Sign and date the plan after updates are made.

- Send a signed, dated copy of all updated plans to the appropriate county emergency management agency (EMA).

- Post the most current emergency plan in a conspicuous location, one that is easy for substitute staff, volunteers, parents, and program licensing/certification inspectors to see.

Date of Incident: _____   Time/Duration of Incident: _____

Brief Description of Incident: _____

_____

Date of the Assessment: _____   Time/Duration of Assessment: _____

Assessor's Organization:				
Address:		City:	State:	Zip:

Assessor's Name:		Phone:	Fax:
		E-mail:	

Name of Facility	**Facility ID**	**Address**	
		STREET	
		CITY	
		COUNTY	ZIP

Name of Director	**Director Cell**	**Alternative Person-in-Charge & Contact Info**		
Facility Contact Details				
PHONE	E-MAIL	FAX	ALTERNATIVE 1	ALTERNATIVE 2

Type of Early Education/Child Care Program

☐ Center   ☐ Accredited Center   ☐ Home-based (family child care or group home)   ☐ Government

☐ Tribal   ☐ Private Nonprofit   ☐ Other   ☐ Not Sure

Type of Insurance

☐ Property   ☐ Hurricane   ☐ Flood (Structure)   ☐ Flood (Contents)   ☐ Tornado   ☐ Other (specify)   ☐ None

What approximate payment is expected from the insurer? _____

Is the building insured to cover the cost of repairs? ☐ Yes   ☐ No

---

Damages

What is your assessment of the damage? ☐ Completely destroyed   ☐ Partially destroyed   ☐ Little or no evidence of damage

Do you have photos of the damages sustained?   ☐ Yes   ☐ No

Is street access available?   ☐ Yes   ☐ No

Were indoor materials damaged or lost?   ☐ Yes   ☐ No

Was outdoor equipment damaged lost?   ☐ Yes   ☐ No

Were appliances damaged or lost?   ☐ Yes   ☐ No

Were stored food, water, and/or other emergency supplies lost?   ☐ Yes   ☐ No

Describe any major EXTERIOR damages such as new or enlarged cracks, broken windows, etc:

Damage/Problem	Location of Damage/Problems	Detailed Descriptions
Main entrance		
Other entrances		
Walls		
Windows		
Roof and/or basement		

Describe any major INTERIOR damages:

Damage/Problem	Location of Damage/Problems	Detailed Descriptions of Damage
Ceiling		
Walls		
Doors		
Floor/Carpet		
Water Leaks		
Toilet		
Light fixtures		
Supplies		
Desks		
Play equipment		

Other useful information:

_____

_____

Employee/Child Status:

	Total #	# Absent	# Injured	# Sent to Hospital	# Dead	# Unaccounted for	# Released to Parents	# Being cared for
Staff								
Children								
Others								

Source of Damage (Check all that apply.)

☐ Flood ☐ Fire ☐ Wind/Wind-driven rain ☐ Earthquake ☐ Other

Estimate of Damages

Repairs	Contents	Total
$	$	$

Operation/Program

Is the facility open? ☐ Yes   ☐ No

If yes, what are the hours of operation? (_____AM/PM — _____AM/PM)

If no, what are the reasons? ☐ Structural damage ☐ No electricity ☐ No water ☐ Flooding

☐ Staff shortage   ☐ Other _____

If no, what are the factors that most impact your ability to reopen?

☐ Return of electricity   ☐ Return of water   ☐ Return of staff

☐ Ability to complete forms to receive assistance

☐ Once forms submitted approval and receive financial assistance

☐ Financial assistance to replace lost or damage materials in classrooms

☐ Families returning to area or enrolling children returning

☐ Other _____

If not open, when is the anticipated reopen date and hours of operation? (Please call back for any future updates.)

Date:_____ (_____AM/PM — _____AM/PM)

If you are currently temporarily closed, are you and/or your staff interested in working in other child care facilities for a limited time?   ☐ Yes   ☐ No

Do you have the capacity to serve additional children? (If you are not at capacity)   ☐ Yes   ☐ No

If yes, how many additional children would you be able to accept? _____

Ages and numbers of additional children who could be accepted:

Infants _____ Toddlers_____ Preschool _____ School-age _____

Do you have a generator system? ☐ Yes   ☐ No   ☐ Working   ☐ Not working

What supplies or materials would you need immediately to continue or resume your program?

Note: This information will be passed onto the emergency management agencies and assistance organizations, but the provision of the items to your sites cannot be guaranteed.

_____

_____

_____

Is the building owned by the agency/organization that operates the program?   ☐ Yes   ☐ No

Is any part of the building rented by the program or any other entity?   ☐ Yes   ☐ No

Is the facility a Head Start program?   ☐ Yes   ☐ No

Does the facility participate in the state child care assistance program?   ☐ Yes   ☐ No

Does the facility participate in the state nutrition program?   ☐ Yes   ☐ No

Number of children served pre-disaster	Number of children served post-disaster (at the time of assessment)
_____ Infants	_____ Infants
_____ Toddlers	_____ Toddlers
_____ Preschoolers	_____ Preschoolers
_____ School-age	_____ School-age

Number of employees pre-disaster _____

Current number of employees (at the time of assessment) _____

Number of employees planning to return to work post-disaster _____

Utility

Is telephone access available at your facility? ☐ Landline   ☐ Cell   ☐ Both   ☐ Neither

Is there electricity available at your facility? ☐ Generator-based   ☐ Normal   ☐ None

Is there water available at your facility? ☐ Normal service   ☐ Bottled   ☐ None

Disaster Applications

Have you completed/submitted a disaster application with FEMA? ☐ Yes   ☐ No

Have you completed/submitted a disaster application with the Small Business Association? ☐ Yes   ☐ No

Other Notes, Comments, Questions That Need to Be Addressed

Adapted with permission from Save the Children. Child Care Initial Rapid Damage Assessment, a tool created by child-focused and emergency management partners in Harris County, TX, including Collaborative for Children, Child Care Licensing, Harris County Office of Homeland Security and Emergency Management, and Save the Children.

Appendix EE

Sample Letter of Agreement With Emergency Evacuation Site

Letter of agreement between _____ and

NAME OF CHILD CARE CENTER

_____ .

NAME OF EMERGENCY EVACUATION SITE

INFORMATION ABOUT CHILD CARE FACILITY	INFORMATION ABOUT EVACUATION SITE
NAME OF FACILITY	NAME OF FACILITY
ADDRESS	ADDRESS
TELEPHONE NUMBER	TELEPHONE NUMBER(S)
NAME OF CONTACT PERSON(S)	NAME OF CONTACT PERSON(S)
HOURS OF OPERATION	HOURS OF OPERATION
NUMBER OF CHILDREN AND STAFF POTENTIALLY EVACUATING	AREA AVAILABLE FOR CENTER OCCUPANCY AT EVACUATION SITE IN SQUARE FEET

Driving directions from child care center to evacuation facility:

_____

_____

_____

_____

_____

(Attach map with directions from child care center to evacuation facility to this agreement.)

Check off items that the evacuation site will provide in an emergency:

☐ Water   ☐ Telephone

☐ Food   ☐ People to assist

☐ Transportation   ☐ Other _____

_____ agrees to serve as an emergency evacuation

NAME OF EVACUATION FACILITY

site for _____

NAME OF CHILD CARE CENTER

Signatures

_____

AUTHORIZED EVACUATION SITE REPRESENTATIVE   DATE

_____

CHILD CARE CENTER DIRECTOR   DATE

Appendix FF

Sample Letter to Parents About Evacuation Arrangements

Date letter distributed: _____

Dear Parents,

Our child care center's philosophy is to keep your child(ren) safe at all times when in our care. With recent world and local events, we have developed an emergency plan that will be put into place in the event that special circumstances require a different type of care. Plans for these special types of care are reviewed annually. Staff members have been instructed about the appropriate response. The local emergency management is aware of these plans. The specific type of emergency will guide where and what special care will be provided.

- **Shelter at the site:** This plan would be put into place in the event of a weather emergency or unsafe outside conditions or threats. In this plan, children will be cared for indoors at the center and the center may be secured or locked to restrict entry. Parents will be notified if they need to pick up their children before their regular time.

- **Evacuation to another site:** This plan would be put into place in the event that it is not safe for the children to remain at the center. In this situation, staff has predetermined alternate sites for care. The choice of site is determined by the specific emergency and what would be an appropriate alternate site.

- **Method to contact parents:** In the event of an emergency, parents will be called, a note will be placed on the door, and radio/TV stations will be alerted to provide more specific information. You can also check for information on our Web site _____ or call our main office at _____ – _____ – _____ . Depending on the distance from the center, the children will walk or be transported to the alternate site.

- **Emergency ends/reuniting with children:** When the emergency ends, parents will be informed and reunited with their children as soon as possible. The contact methods listed above will be used to inform parents.

The purpose for sharing this information with you is not to cause you worry but to reassure you that we are prepared to handle all types of emergencies in a way that will ensure the safety of your child(ren). In the event of an actual emergency, please do not call the center—it will be important to keep the lines open. If you have questions regarding this information, talk with the center director or your child's teacher.

Sincerely,

_____
SIGNATURE OF CHILD CARE CENTER DIRECTOR

This sample letter may be downloaded from www.betterkidcare.psu.edu/page14.html.

Appendix GG

Evacuation Drill Log

Select a location in the building for the site of a pretend fire and other types of hazards that would change the usual emergency procedure. Plan and conduct an emergency drill varying the type and location of the emergency.

Date	Time	Pretend Fire or Hazard Type and Location	Length of Time to Evacuate/ Shelter in Place/Lockdown	Number of Children	Name/Signature of Person Observing Drill

Appendix HH

What Is Child Abuse and Neglect? Recognizing the Signs and Symptoms

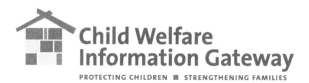

Child Welfare Information Gateway

PROTECTING CHILDREN ■ STRENGTHENING FAMILIES

FACTSHEET

July 2013

Disponible en español
https://www.childwelfare.gov/
pubs/factsheets/ques.cfm

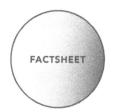

What Is Child Abuse and Neglect? Recognizing the Signs and Symptoms

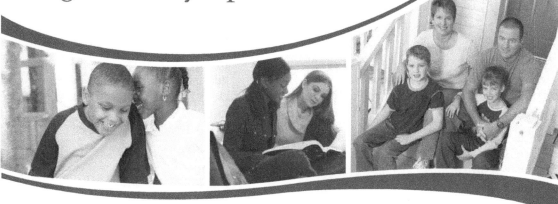

The first step in helping abused or neglected children is learning to recognize the signs of child abuse and neglect. The presence of a single sign does not mean that child maltreatment is occurring in a family, but a closer look at the situation may be warranted when these signs appear repeatedly or in combination. This factsheet is intended to help you better understand the legal definition of child abuse and neglect, learn about the different types

What's Inside:

- How is child abuse and neglect defined in Federal law?
- What are the major types of child abuse and neglect?
- Recognizing signs of abuse and neglect
- Resources

Use your smartphone to access this factsheet online.

Children's Bureau

Child Welfare Information Gateway
Children's Bureau/ACYF/ACF/HHS
1250 Maryland Avenue, SW
Eighth Floor
Washington, DC 20024
800.394.3366
Email: info@childwelfare.gov
https://www.childwelfare.gov

of abuse and neglect, and recognize the signs and symptoms of abuse and neglect. Resources about the impact of trauma on well-being also are included in this factsheet.

How Is Child Abuse and Neglect Defined in Federal Law?

Federal legislation lays the groundwork for State laws on child maltreatment by identifying a minimum set of acts or behaviors that define child abuse and neglect. The Federal Child Abuse Prevention and Treatment Act (CAPTA), (42 U.S.C.A. §5106g), as amended and reauthorized by the CAPTA Reauthorization Act of 2010, defines child abuse and neglect as, at minimum:

"Any recent act or failure to act on the part of a parent or caretaker which results in death, serious physical or emotional harm, sexual abuse or exploitation; or an act or failure to act which presents an imminent risk of serious harm."

Most Federal and State child protection laws primarily refer to cases of harm to a child caused by parents or other caregivers; they generally do not include harm caused by other people, such as acquaintances or strangers. Some State laws also include a child's witnessing of domestic violence as a form of abuse or neglect.

CHILD ABUSE AND NEGLECT STATISTICS

- *Child Maltreatment*
  This report summarizes annual child abuse statistics submitted by States to the National Child Abuse and Neglect Data System (NCANDS). It includes information about child maltreatment reports, victims, fatalities, perpetrators, services, and additional research:
  http://www.acf.hhs.gov/programs/cb/research-data-technology/statistics-research/child-maltreatment

- Child Welfare Outcomes Report Data
  This website provides information on the performance of States in seven outcome categories related to the safety, permanency, and well-being of children involved in the child welfare system. Data, which are made available on the website prior to the release of the annual report, include the number of child victims of maltreatment:
  http://cwoutcomes.acf.hhs.gov/data/overview

What Are the Major Types of Child Abuse and Neglect?

Within the minimum standards set by CAPTA, each State is responsible for providing its own definitions of child abuse and neglect. Most States recognize the four major types of maltreatment: physical abuse, neglect, sexual abuse, and emotional abuse. Signs and symptoms for each type of maltreatment are listed below. Additionally, many States identify abandonment and parental substance abuse as abuse or neglect. While these types of maltreatment may be found separately, they often occur in combination. For State-specific laws pertaining to child abuse and neglect, see Child Welfare Information Gateway's State Statutes Search page: https://www.childwelfare.gov/systemwide/laws_policies/state/

Information Gateway's *Definitions of Child Abuse and Neglect* provides civil definitions that determine the grounds for intervention by State child protective agencies: https://www.childwelfare.gov/systemwide/laws_policies/statutes/define.pdf

Physical abuse is nonaccidental physical injury (ranging from minor bruises to severe fractures or death) as a result of punching, beating, kicking, biting, shaking, throwing, stabbing, choking, hitting (with a hand, stick, strap, or other object), burning, or otherwise harming a child, that is inflicted by a parent, caregiver, or other person who

has responsibility for the child.[1] Such injury is considered abuse regardless of whether the caregiver intended to hurt the child. Physical discipline, such as spanking or paddling, is not considered abuse as long as it is reasonable and causes no bodily injury to the child.

Neglect is the failure of a parent, guardian, or other caregiver to provide for a child's basic needs. Neglect may be:

- Physical (e.g., failure to provide necessary food or shelter, or lack of appropriate supervision)

- Medical (e.g., failure to provide necessary medical or mental health treatment)[2]

- Educational (e.g., failure to educate a child or attend to special education needs)

- Emotional (e.g., inattention to a child's emotional needs, failure to provide psychological care, or permitting the child to use alcohol or other drugs)

Sometimes cultural values, the standards of care in the community, and poverty may contribute to maltreatment, indicating

---

[1] Nonaccidental injury that is inflicted by someone other than a parent, guardian, relative, or other caregiver (i.e., a stranger), is considered a criminal act that is not addressed by child protective services.

[2] *Withholding of medically indicated treatment* is a specific form of medical neglect that is defined by CAPTA as "the failure to respond to the infant's life-threatening conditions by providing treatment (including appropriate nutrition, hydration, and medication) which, in the treating physician's or physicians' reasonable medical judgment, will be most likely to be effective in ameliorating or correcting all such conditions..." CAPTA does note a few exceptions, including infants who are "chronically and irreversibly comatose"; situations when providing treatment would not save the infant's life but merely prolong dying; or when "the provision of such treatment would be virtually futile in terms of the survival of the infant and the treatment itself under such circumstances would be inhumane."

the family is in need of information or assistance. When a family fails to use information and resources, and the child's health or safety is at risk, then child welfare intervention may be required. In addition, many States provide an exception to the definition of neglect for parents who choose not to seek medical care for their children due to religious beliefs.[3]

Sexual abuse includes activities by a parent or caregiver such as fondling a child's genitals, penetration, incest, rape, sodomy, indecent exposure, and exploitation through prostitution or the production of pornographic materials.

Sexual abuse is defined by CAPTA as "the employment, use, persuasion, inducement, enticement, or coercion of any child to engage in, or assist any other person to engage in, any sexually explicit conduct or simulation of such conduct for the purpose of producing a visual depiction of such conduct; or the rape, and in cases of caretaker or inter-familial relationships, statutory rape, molestation, prostitution, or other form of sexual exploitation of children, or incest with children."

Emotional abuse (or psychological abuse) is a pattern of behavior that impairs a child's emotional development or sense of self-worth. This may include constant criticism, threats, or rejection, as well as withholding love, support, or guidance. Emotional abuse is often difficult to prove, and therefore, child protective services may not be able to intervene without evidence of harm or

mental injury to the child. Emotional abuse is almost always present when other types of maltreatment are identified.

Abandonment is now defined in many States as a form of neglect. In general, a child is considered to be abandoned when the parent's identity or whereabouts are unknown, the child has been left alone in circumstances where the child suffers serious harm, or the parent has failed to maintain contact with the child or provide reasonable support for a specified period of time. Some States have enacted laws—often called safe haven laws—that provide safe places for parents to relinquish newborn infants. Child Welfare Information Gateway produced a publication as part of its State Statute series that summarizes such State laws. *Infant Safe Haven Laws* is available on the Information Gateway website: https://www.childwelfare.gov/systemwide/laws_policies/statutes/safehaven.cfm

Substance abuse is an element of the definition of child abuse or neglect in many States. Circumstances that are considered abuse or neglect in some States include the following:

- Prenatal exposure of a child to harm due to the mother's use of an illegal drug or other substance

- Manufacture of methamphetamine in the presence of a child

- Selling, distributing, or giving illegal drugs or alcohol to a child

- Use of a controlled substance by a caregiver that impairs the caregiver's ability to adequately care for the child

---

[3] The CAPTA amendments of 1996 (42 U.S.C.A. § 5106i) added new provisions specifying that nothing in the act be construed as establishing a Federal requirement that a parent or legal guardian provide any medical service or treatment that is against the religious beliefs of the parent or legal guardian.

For more information about this issue, see Child Welfare Information Gateway's *Parental Drug Use as Child Abuse* at https://www.childwelfare.gov/systemwide/laws_policies/statutes/drugexposed.cfm

Recognizing Signs of Abuse and Neglect

In addition to working to prevent a child from experiencing abuse or neglect, it is important to recognize high-risk situations and the signs and symptoms of maltreatment. If you do suspect a child is being harmed, reporting your suspicions may protect him or her and get help for the family. Any concerned person can report suspicions of child abuse or neglect. Reporting your concerns is not making an accusation; rather, it is a request for an investigation and assessment to determine if help is needed.

Some people (typically certain types of professionals, such as teachers or physicians) are required by State law to make a report of child maltreatment under specific circumstances—these are called mandatory reporters. Some States require all adults to report suspicions of child abuse or neglect. Child Welfare Information Gateway's publication *Mandatory Reporters of Child Abuse and Neglect* discusses the laws that designate groups of professionals as mandatory reporters: https://www.childwelfare.gov/systemwide/laws_policies/statutes/manda.cfm

For information about where and how to file a report, contact your local child protective services agency or police department.

Childhelp National Child Abuse Hotline (800.4.A.CHILD) and its website offer crisis intervention, information, resources, and referrals to support services and provide assistance in 170 languages: http://www.childhelp.org/pages/hotline-home

For information on what happens when suspected abuse or neglect is reported, read Information Gateway's *How the Child Welfare System Works*: https://www.childwelfare.gov/pubs/factsheets/cpswork.pdf

Some children may directly disclose that they have experienced abuse or neglect. The factsheet *How to Handle Child Abuse Disclosures*, produced by the "Childhelp Speak Up Be Safe" child abuse prevention campaign, offers tips. The factsheet defines direct and indirect disclosure, as well as tips for supporting the child: http://www.speakupbesafe.org/parents/disclosures-for-parents.pdf

The following signs may signal the presence of child abuse or neglect.

The Child:

- Shows sudden changes in behavior or school performance

- Has not received help for physical or medical problems brought to the parents' attention

- Has learning problems (or difficulty concentrating) that cannot be attributed to specific physical or psychological causes

- Is always watchful, as though preparing for something bad to happen

- Lacks adult supervision

- Is overly compliant, passive, or withdrawn

- Comes to school or other activities early, stays late, and does not want to go home

- Is reluctant to be around a particular person

- Discloses maltreatment

The Parent:

- Denies the existence of—or blames the child for—the child's problems in school or at home

- Asks teachers or other caregivers to use harsh physical discipline if the child misbehaves

- Sees the child as entirely bad, worthless, or burdensome

- Demands a level of physical or academic performance the child cannot achieve

- Looks primarily to the child for care, attention, and satisfaction of the parent's emotional needs

- Shows little concern for the child

The Parent and Child:

- Rarely touch or look at each other

- Consider their relationship entirely negative

- State that they do not like each other

The above list may not be *all* the signs of abuse or neglect. It is important to pay attention to other behaviors that may seem unusual or concerning. In addition to these signs and symptoms, Child Welfare Information Gateway provides information on the risk factors and perpetrators of child abuse and neglect fatalities: https://www.childwelfare.gov/can/risk_perpetrators.cfm

Signs of Physical Abuse

Consider the possibility of physical abuse when the **child:**

- Has unexplained burns, bites, bruises, broken bones, or black eyes

- Has fading bruises or other marks noticeable after an absence from school

- Seems frightened of the parents and protests or cries when it is time to go home

- Shrinks at the approach of adults

- Reports injury by a parent or another adult caregiver

- Abuses animals or pets

Consider the possibility of physical abuse when the **parent or other adult caregiver:**

- Offers conflicting, unconvincing, or no explanation for the child's injury, or provides an explanation that is not consistent with the injury

- Describes the child as "evil" or in some other very negative way

- Uses harsh physical discipline with the child

- Has a history of abuse as a child

- Has a history of abusing animals or pets

Signs of Neglect

Consider the possibility of neglect when the **child:**

- Is frequently absent from school

- Begs or steals food or money

- Lacks needed medical or dental care, immunizations, or glasses

- Is consistently dirty and has severe body odor

- Lacks sufficient clothing for the weather

- Abuses alcohol or other drugs

- States that there is no one at home to provide care

Consider the possibility of neglect when the **parent or other adult caregiver:**

- Appears to be indifferent to the child

- Seems apathetic or depressed

- Behaves irrationally or in a bizarre manner

- Is abusing alcohol or other drugs

Signs of Sexual Abuse

Consider the possibility of sexual abuse when the **child:**

- Has difficulty walking or sitting

- Suddenly refuses to change for gym or to participate in physical activities

- Reports nightmares or bedwetting

- Experiences a sudden change in appetite

- Demonstrates bizarre, sophisticated, or unusual sexual knowledge or behavior

- Becomes pregnant or contracts a venereal disease, particularly if under age 14

- Runs away

- Reports sexual abuse by a parent or another adult caregiver

- Attaches very quickly to strangers or new adults in their environment

Consider the possibility of sexual abuse when the **parent or other adult caregiver:**

- Is unduly protective of the child or severely limits the child's contact with other children, especially of the opposite sex

- Is secretive and isolated

- Is jealous or controlling with family members

Signs of Emotional Maltreatment

Consider the possibility of emotional maltreatment when the **child:**

- Shows extremes in behavior, such as overly compliant or demanding behavior, extreme passivity, or aggression

- Is either inappropriately adult (parenting other children, for example) or inappropriately infantile (frequently rocking or head-banging, for example)

- Is delayed in physical or emotional development

- Has attempted suicide

- Reports a lack of attachment to the parent

Consider the possibility of emotional maltreatment when the **parent or other adult caregiver:**

- Constantly blames, belittles, or berates the child

- Is unconcerned about the child and refuses to consider offers of help for the child's problems

- Overtly rejects the child

THE IMPACT OF CHILDHOOD TRAUMA ON WELL-BEING

Child abuse and neglect can have lifelong implications for victims, including on their well-being. While the physical wounds heal, there are several long-term consequences of experiencing the trauma of abuse or neglect. A child or youth's ability to cope and even thrive after trauma is called "resilience," and with help, many of these children can work through and overcome their past experiences.

Children who are maltreated often are at risk of experiencing cognitive delays and emotional difficulties, among other issues. Childhood trauma also negatively affects nervous system and immune system development, putting children who have been maltreated at a higher risk for health problems as adults. For more information on the lasting effects of child abuse and neglect, read Child Welfare Information Gateway's factsheet *Long-Term Consequences of Child Abuse and Neglect*: https://www.childwelfare.gov/pubs/factsheets/long_term_consequences.cfm

The National Child Traumatic Stress Network's webpage What Is Child Traumatic Stress offers definitions, materials on understanding child traumatic stress, and several Q&A documents: http://www.nctsn.org/resources/audiences/parents-caregivers/what-is-cts

The Monique Burr Foundation for Children's brief *Speak Up Be Safe: The Impact of Child Abuse and Neglect* explains the immediate and long-term consequences of child abuse and neglect to child, family, school, and community well-being: http://www.moniqueburrfoundation.org/SUBS/Resources/Impact_of_Abuse_and_Neglect.pdf

The National Council for Adoption's article "Supporting Maltreated Children: Countering the Effects of Neglect and Abuse" explains several issues common to children that have experienced abuse or neglect and offers suggestions for parents and caregivers on talking with children and helping them overcome past traumas: https://www.adoptioncouncil.org/images/stories/documents/NCFA_ADOPTION_ADVOCATE_NO48.pdf

ZERO TO THREE produced *Building Resilience: The Power to Cope With Adversity*, which presents tips and strategies for helping families and children build resilience after trauma: http://www.zerotothree.org/maltreatment/31-1-prac-tips-beardslee.pdf

Resources

Child Welfare Information Gateway's web section on child abuse and neglect provides information on identifying abuse, statistics, risk and protective factors, and more: https://www.childwelfare.gov/can/

The Information Gateway Reporting Child Abuse and Neglect webpage provides information about mandatory reporting and how to report suspected abuse: https://www.childwelfare.gov/responding/reporting.cfm

The National Child Abuse Prevention Month web section provides tip sheets for parents and caregivers, available in English and Spanish, that focus on concrete strategies for taking care of children and strengthening families: https://www.childwelfare.gov/preventing/preventionmonth/tipsheets.cfm

Information Gateway also has produced a number of publications about child abuse and neglect:

- *Child Maltreatment: Past, Present, and Future:* https://www.childwelfare.gov/pubs/issue_briefs/cm_prevention.pdf

- *Long-Term Consequences of Child Abuse and Neglect:* https://www.childwelfare.gov/pubs/factsheets/long_term_consequences.pdf

- *Preventing Child Abuse and Neglect:* https://www.childwelfare.gov/pubs/factsheets/preventingcan.pdf

- *Understanding the Effects of Maltreatment on Brain Development:* https://www.childwelfare.gov/pubs/issue_briefs/brain_development/brain_development.pdf

The Centers for Disease Control and Prevention (CDC) produced *Understanding Child Maltreatment*, which defines the many types of maltreatment and the CDC's approach to prevention, in addition to providing additional resources: http://www.cdc.gov/violenceprevention/pdf/cm_factsheet2012-a.pdf

Prevent Child Abuse America is a national organization dedicated to providing information on child maltreatment and its prevention: http://www.preventchildabuse.org/index.shtml

The National Child Traumatic Stress Network strives to raise the standard of care and improve access to services for traumatized children, their families, and communities: http://www.nctsn.org/

Stand for Children advocates for improvements to, and funding for, programs that give every child a fair chance in life: http://stand.org/

A list of organizations focused on child maltreatment prevention is available in Information Gateway's National Child Abuse Prevention Partner Organizations page: https://www.childwelfare.gov/pubs/reslist/rl_dsp.cfm?rs_id=21&rate_chno=19-00044

Acknowledgment:

This updated factsheet is based on a previous publication that was adapted, with permission, from *Recognizing Child Abuse: What Parents Should Know.* Prevent Child Abuse America. ©2003.

Suggested Citation:

Child Welfare Information Gateway. (2013). *What is child abuse and neglect? Recognizing the signs and symptoms.* Washington, DC: U.S. Department of Health and Human Services, Children's Bureau.

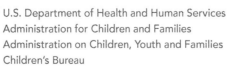 U.S. Department of Health and Human Services
Administration for Children and Families
Administration on Children, Youth and Families
Children's Bureau

 ACF

 Children's Bureau

Index

Toilets
  adaption for independent use, 44
  equipment in, 45
  location of, 44
  maintenance of, 45
Tooth decay
  from drinking milk, 28
  emergencies, 73
  prevention of, 67
Toothbrushing procedures, 72
Toxic substances. *See also* Prohibited substances
  in art supplies, 56
  in furnishings, 55
  lead, 57–58
  for maintenance, 53
  mercury, 58
  mold, 54
  pesticides, 52–53
  plants, 56
  in play areas, 58
  protection from, 105
  safety checks for, 59–60
  sand, 56
  secondhand smoke, 105
  in sensory materials, 56
  storage of, 114
  in toys, 54
  use of, 114
Toxicity, definition of, 51
Toys
  cleaning of, 46, 60, Appendix U-173–174
  lead in, 58
  safety checks for, 59–60
  toxicity of, 54
Training. *See also* Professional development
  care of children with special needs, 3, 74, 111, Appendix
      G-137–141, Appendix H-143–146
  child abuse and neglect protection, 103, Appendix
      HH-207–216
  child passenger safety, 65
  drivers, 6–62
  emergencies, 91–92, 100
  feeding children, 30
  first aid and CPR, 91–92, 110
  food service, 30, 111
  integrated pest management, 53
  medication administration, 75–76, Appendix X-179–183
  ongoing professional development, 110
  pesticide operators, 53
  preservice, 110
  related to performance reviews, 110
  stress from lack of, Appendix V-175
  transportation, 65
  volunteers and substitutes, 10
  water safety, 110
Transitions plans, 18

Transportation. *See also* Motor vehicles
  allowable times for, 64
  arrangements for emergencies, Appendix F-136
  bicycles, 66
  to emergency facilities, 93
  procedures of
      drop-off and pickup, 63
      passenger safety, 63–64
      specialized training for, 65
      walking safety, 65–66
  wheelchair, 64
Tuberculosis (TB) screening, 70

U
Ultraviolet (UV) radiation, 34, 57

V
Vaccine Education Center at Children's Hospital of Philadelphia,
      Appendix E-131
Vaccine refusal, 4, Appendix E-129–132
Vaccines. *See* Immunizations
Vehicles. *See* Motor vehicles
Ventilation standards, 51
Volunteers, 10

W
Washing. *See also* Hand washing
  bottles, 28
  dishes, 25
  hand, 40
  toys, 46, 60
Water
  availability of, 20
  fluoride in, 72
  lead in, 57
  supply, 54
Water play
  communal, 54
  equipment, 46
  gross motor, 11
Water safety training, 110
Weapons, prohibition of, 106
Weather, 33–34
Wheelchair transport, 64
Why Immunize?, Appendix E-131